KU-452-052

# Primal Health

# PRIMAL HEALTH

A Blueprint for Our Survival

*Michel Odent*

THE BRITISH SCHOOL OF OSTEOPATHY
1-4 SUFFOLK ST., LONDON. SW1Y 4HG
TEL. 01-930 9254-8

CENTURY
LONDON MELBOURNE AUCKLAND JOHANNESBURG

Copyright © Michel Odent 1986

*All rights reserved*

First published in 1986 by Century Hutchinson Ltd,
Brookmount House, 62–65 Chandos Place, Covent Garden,
London WC2N 4NW

Century Hutchinson Publishing Group (Australia) Pty Ltd,
16–22 Church Street, Hawthorn, Melbourne, Victoria 3122

Century Hutchinson Group (NZ) Ltd,
32–34 View Road, PO Box 40–086, Glenfield, Auckland 10

Century Hutchinson Group (SA) Pty Ltd,
PO Box 337, Bergvlei 2012, South Africa

Phototypeset in Linotron Plantin by
Input Typesetting Ltd, London SW19 8DR

Printed in Great Britain by
St Edmundsbury Press Ltd, Bury St Edmunds, Suffolk
Bound by Butler & Tanner Ltd, Frome, Somerset

British Library Cataloguing in Publication Data

Odent, Michel
  Primal health: a blueprint for our
  survival.
  1. Natural childbirth
  I. Title
  618.4′5        RC.661

  ISBN 0–7126–1268–8

This book is dedicated to Antoine Béchamp.
Why Antoine Béchamp?
Not because he understood the mechanism of
fermentation before Pasteur.
Not because he knew about germs before Pasteur.
Not because he demonstrated the role of micro-organisms
in certain diseases.
*But* because, in the euphoria of Pasteur's glory, he dared
to say:
'Instead of trying to determine what abnormal conditions
disease is composed of, let us first know the normal
conditions which make us healthy.'

# Acknowledgements

I would like to thank the people who helped me to understand the true meaning of the word 'primal', from William Shakespeare to Arthur Janov.

'My offence hath the primall eldest curse upon't, A brother's murther'

William Shakespeare

'The Primal Scream'

Arthur Janov

My thanks to Pascal, born while I was writing this book and to his wonderful mother Judy. Both of them are my teachers in primal health.

# Contents

# Linguistic Note

This book has been written in English and French simultaneously. Because there is no equivalent, certain English words have not been translated. The word 'primal', meaning first in time and first in importance, does not have a corresponding translation in French. I was also unable to find a French word which expressed with every shade and nuance the terms 'hopelessness' and 'helplessness'.

In the same way, I have used certain French words and expressions in the English edition without trying to translate them. The first such word is *terrain*. The original meaning of *terrain* is soil, but in my text I have used it to mean the basic condition, the temperament, the ability to cope with disease.

I have also been unable to translate the exact meaning of the phrase *prise de conscience*. *Prise de conscience* has something to do with consciousness-raising. It means something like 'sudden new awareness', although this phrase does not exactly capture the unexpectedness of the flash of awareness.

Throughout the book I have tried to keep the medical terminology as simple as possible. However in order to help the general reader, I have printed a Glossary at the end of the book to explain in greater detail the more important medical terms which have to be grasped before the concept of primal health can be fully understood.

# CHAPTER 1

# What is Health?

We are in the nursery of a big maternity unit in Eastern Europe where several dozen newborn babies are arranged side by side, all of them wrapped in swaddling. Regularly, at a precise time, a nurse wearing a mask conscientiously obeys her orders and goes to fetch one of the little parcels. It is feeding time.

This experience left me feeling that something was wrong. I felt these babies were in danger. I knew that these newborn babies were already beginning to lose that impulse which makes us struggle, struggle for life. This knowledge didn't come to me from reading books, nor from any process of reasoning. It came more directly, from the emotions. And feeling emotions is a way of knowing.

After I came back from my trip in the late 1970s, I couldn't stop thinking about the babies in that nursery. I asked myself what beliefs, what theories, what principles could possibly explain why those babies were separated from their mothers, thus learning that it is useless to cry, useless to ask for anything, useless to express their needs in any way at all? On the face of it, it's done in the name of science. Those babies were entrusted to medicine, which considers itself to be scientific. Science has taught us that germs are dangerous, and has calculated the nutritional needs of babies. So, in the name of science, those babies were protected from family germs, and at the same time guaranteed the ideal amount of food. Since medicine pretends to be ruled by science and since these days babies belong to medicine, let us then use science to suggest that many babies are in danger.

While I was thinking about these newborn babies, the true significance of some very well-known experiments suddenly dawned on me. These experiments, with dogs or rats, showed how animals can learn to be helpless. During the 1960s, Martin Seligman and his colleagues conducted a series of experiments to test a learning theory. They divided some dogs into two groups. The first group was given electric shocks from which they could do absolutely nothing to escape. The second group of dogs was placed in identical cages, but given no shocks at all.

The same two groups of dogs were then tested in a special box which had two compartments divided by a barrier. In one compartment, the dogs received an electric shock. But by jumping over the barrier, they could escape the shocks. The second group of dogs, which had never had any electric shocks before, very quickly discovered the escape route and jumped over the barrier. But the astounding thing was that the first group of dogs – those which had previously been shocked – did not make any attempt to escape. They just crouched helplessly in the electric shock compartment. Even when the dogs were lifted over the barrier to the safe side, it still made no difference. They had learned from their first experience that nothing they did made any difference, and they were unable to control events. Seligman called this behaviour 'learned helplessness'.

Later, other researchers wanted to find out what physiological changes would occur in rats when they were given varying degrees of control over electric shocks. They found that when the rats had no control over the shocks, they suffered stomach ulcers and weight loss. These rats also had lower levels of adrenalin, the hormone which gives sudden energy to be able to fight, or to run away. The rats were not made ill by the electric shocks, but by the state of submission they were in at the time of the shocks.

In France, Henri Laborit was another scientist who studied the effects of unavoidable electric shocks. What he found was that if a pair of rats were put together in a cage while receiving electric shocks, they were protected against a rise in blood pressure by fighting each other. But the rats which could neither fight nor run away did suffer a rise in blood pressure. Laborit coined the phrase 'inhibition of action'. This is both a behavioural and a hormonal response; in particular it affects the secretion of hormones which depress the immune system. This is the system which enables the body to recognize foreign substances and to fight against such invaders as bacteria, viruses, parasites, cancerous cells, and so on.

The implications of all these basic experiments are of paramount importance. They help us to understand just how much a person's entire capabilities are decreased when they have no control over what happens to them, and can only passively submit. They also help us to understand that the responses of the nervous system, the hormonal system and the immune system should never be disassociated. They form a whole.

Thus it was that my first thoughts about life for a newborn baby in a nursery led me to what scientists say about 'submissive behaviour'. In fact, these thoughts could just as well have led me to what they say about the process of attachment between mother and baby, or the importance of sensory stimulation during infancy. No matter, as all these are just different approaches to the same truth. Modern science is moving ahead so fast now that it can even explain, in a variety of ways, that a newborn baby needs its mother!

11

The example I have chosen of how I felt after visiting that nursery is just one amongst countless others. For every day a doctor's life is enriched by new feelings and sudden *prises de conscience* (*see* Linguistic note, p. 8). Practising surgery, whether it's war or civilian surgery, you're always confronted with the struggle to survive, or else the recovery of a particular function. You're sometimes confronted with death.

In my own experience, however, it is birth scenes which leave the greatest mark. Being present at the birth of thousands of babies changes you into a different person – as long as the births are not too disturbed by the medical establishment. The holy atmosphere of a birthing room is catching. And to share this holy atmosphere gives you a more global vision. It helps you sort out the essential from matters of secondary importance. When you are in a birthing place, you learn to put aside the analytical functions of the brain. During the period of my life when I was most involved in birth, I noticed that I was better able to ignore certain established ideas. Little by little, I began to look at things in a very personal way. A good example of this is my way of understanding the word 'health'.

Amongst doctors, the word health usually means the absence of disease. As early as the sixteenth century, the French author Montaigne said that doctors are governed by disease. The mental image associated with the word disease is still not very different from the traditional image of the demon invading the ill person's body; the demon has to be driven out before the sick person can be healed. Disease is something which can be got rid of, rather than something which is part and parcel of the whole person. The idea of health as the absence of disease is based on an old myth which says that each disease has its own cause, and therefore has its own specific treatment. For example, discovering a virus as the cause of a particular disease is a perfect example of this way of looking at things.

While this mental image is still prevalent in the medical world, other images of health have been gaining ground amongst the general public. As soon as you mention the word health, people think straightaway of good nutrition, exercise, relaxation and lifestyle in general. But this commonly heard association of ideas is actually no more helpful in defining the real nature of good health. Certainly, good nutrition, exercise and positive emotions are good advice to anyone who wants to maintain or cultivate what they already have. But it is impossible to make any radical change in the way our biological computers have been programmed at the primal period of life.

Health cannot really be understood outside the context of the struggle for life. There is no life without struggle. You cannot explain life by the laws of physics alone. Life itself is a constant struggle against one of the fundamental laws of physics: the tendency of energy to become less available to do work with the passing of time – what is commonly called 'entropy'. If you think about any aspect of life, it is impossible to disassociate it from the concept of struggle. Take, for example, the evolution of the species, and immediately we find the concepts of selection and competition, in other words the concept of struggle.

There is a permanent struggle between different species before an ecological harmony can be reached and maintained. Even within a particular species, sexual rivalry is a way for individual members to strive for survival through their own offspring, by transmitting their own genes. Love, attachment, fellowship within one species, or even between species, may be considered to be a part of a strategy to reinforce the capacity to struggle. Even if we take the most sophisticated aspects of life – human societies – we see that the early theorists of social change soon discovered the importance of class struggles.

What, then, is the place of health among the different aspects of the struggle for life?

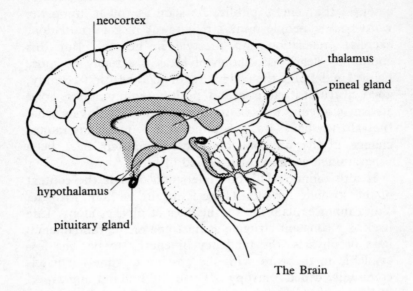

neocortex

thalamus

pineal gland

hypothalamus

pituitary gland

The Brain

Health is a system which allows us to struggle on a minute-to-minute basis and to adapt constantly to the environment. This system has an orchestrator. Not to know its name and role is a bit like discussing politics in the USA without knowing about the White House. It belongs to the most archaic, primitive structures of the brain; to that part of the brain which dates back to the ancient history of life. It is the conductor of health in all mammals, and in humans in particular. It is called the hypothalamus.

The role of the hypothalamus as the regulator of hunger, thirst and sexual rhythms has been well known for decades. But it is only recently that its paramount importance has been understood. The hypothalamus has a close relationship with other structures of the brain as well as with the autonomous nervous system. That is why I use the less precise concept of 'primal brain' to cover the hypothalamus and its associated structures (see Glossary, p. 163).

The primal brain controls the hormonal secretions of different endocrine glands. In fact, the brain itself could be considered as a gland since the hypothalamus secretes hormones, and since the nerve cells communicate between themselves by chemical messengers which are not very different from hormones. So any distinction between the primal brain and the hormonal system is now obsolete. In the same way, all traditional divisions between the primal brain and the immune system are also obsolete. There are no divisions. The word health means the way our 'primal adaptive system' works as a whole (see Glossary, p. 163).

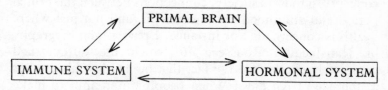

The primal adaptive system is a whole.

Certain situations trigger a sudden change in the workings of the primal adaptive system. Imagine yourself in two different situations: you have won the pools, or a burglar is threatening you with a gun. It makes no difference whether the feeling is one of joy or fear. Whenever emotions are felt, there is a response by the entire primal adaptive system. So there is a response in the brain, the immune system and the hormonal system, all in unison.

It is during fetal life, the time around birth and infancy that the different parts of this system develop and regulate and adjust themselves. At the end of infancy, the primal adaptive system has reached maturity. I call primal health the balancing of the set point levels (see Glossary, p. 164) which have been reached by the end of infancy. To understand what set point levels mean, think of a central heating thermostat. You set the thermostat to a particular temperature at the beginning of the day, and the heating reaches the temperature you have set. It is similar with our hormonal levels, which have to be set at the beginning of life and which continue to 'switch on' at the set level. Thus, primal health is built at that time when the baby is closely dependent on its mother, first in the womb, then during childbirth, and then during the period of breastfeeding. Everything which happens during this period of dependence on the mother has an influence on this basic state of health, this primal health.

There are many things which lead me to believe that the way I perceive health is radically different from the usual concept. In today's society, connections between the primal period and adulthood are uncommon, and not just where health is concerned. For instance, I read a long biography of Jean-Jacques Rousseau in which the author had completely overlooked the fact that he had lost his mother at the age of ten days! When people do attempt to make these connections, it is only because they are interested in sensory functions. They might ask questions like what can a baby perceive in the womb? Or, what can a newborn baby see? But obviously they are more interested in learning capabilities than in health as a whole.

It seems to be not yet well understood that a sensory function at the beginning of life can be a means of stimulating the primal brain at a time when the primal adaptive system has not yet reached full maturity. In simple terms it means that when, for example, you caress a human baby or the young of any animal you are also stimulating its immune system. The knowledge of the universe which we have through our sensory organs takes us on to another aspect of the struggle for life, which is outside the field of health.

The mental imagery commonly associated with the word health is in itself dangerous and life-destroying. The concept of primal health might make it easier to shift our priorities and to rediscover the fundamental needs which a human being has at the beginning of his life. My understanding the word health might have huge practical consequences. After all, to a great extent the world is governed by words.

# CHAPTER 2

# The Primal Adaptive System

The newboy syndrome at college is universally known. During the first weeks, newcomers share a particular emotional state. According to serious scientific and medical literature, new students have a high level of cortisol and their immune system is disturbed at the start of their first year. Similarly, studies of groups of men have shown them to have a very specific hormonal state and depressed immune systems six weeks after the death of their spouse. It is something totally new to be able to say that a particular emotional state is always associated with both a specific hormonal state and with a reaction in the immune system.

The deeper I go into the spectacular breakthroughs of the biological sciences, the more my views are reinforced. If all this new data were to be incorporated, it would help us reach a new vision of life, particularly of the human phenomenon. But dividing the different disciplines, and putting them into separate compartments, makes this synthesis difficult. For example, I know a recent book about immunology in which you cannot find the word hypothalamus! I have also noticed that the immune system does not get so much as a mention in certain recent well-known books on the brain and nervous system.

So the first thing we have to do is to smash the barriers between these disciplines. They get in the way. We have to show that the barriers are artificial, and get us nowhere. Smashing barriers is an essential first step before the word health can be truly understood, and before defining the primal adaptive system. I also want to show that the different parts of this system mature very early in life, at the time when the baby is dependent on the mother. In this respect, the primal adaptive system is totally different from the 'new brain' or neocortex, which can increase its capacity until a very advanced age if it is stimulated enough (see p. 29).

## The Immune System – A Reminder

First of all, everyone interested in health should keep in mind some basic facts about what we call the immune system. It plays a key role in many modern diseases, as for example, in the mysterious AIDS – Acquired Immune Deficiency Syndrome – about which the news media have stirred up a lot of fear and curiosity. For anyone not familiar with the biological sciences, there follow some key words which should help explain how the immune system works. This reminder about the immune system will also give me a chance to break through another barrier – the barrier of language. It will also reinforce the idea that life is a constant struggle between ourselves and the environment.

To make the immune system easier to understand, I shall play toy soldiers and use military language. The immune system is the body's defence system, the means by which it fights off potentially dangerous foreign organisms such as bacteria. From the moment we are born, we live among bacteria. We need bacteria. But in some circumstances certain bacteria can be dangerous and must be fought off. The first line of defence is the *frontier*, such as the skin or the mucous membrane, which bacteria cannot easily get through. If an entry gate is open, such as a small wound, *the frontier guards* will organize *local resistance*, no matter who the invaders are. This is called inflammation. *The local battleground* is red, hot and painful because more blood reaches the area. Mobile white blood cells called phagocytes arrive on the scene as reinforcements and join in the local fight, encircling the bacteria and destroying them. The usual outcome is a rapid and complete victory for the defending army. Sometimes, however, victory is only possible with the formation of pus, which means the destruction of many white cells and phagocytes. In some cases, the local defence is overcome and the battle moves to the lymphatic nodes or to organs such as the liver, spleen or lungs. If there is a repeated penetration of bacteria into the bloodstream, it is called septicemia. Total *defeat* of the body's defences is possible. Resistance to invaders can be reinforced by an acquired immunity. The immune system can learn: it has a memory. It has to learn how to fight specific enemies by using billions of different types of antibodies. These antibodies *patrol* and protect the body and are made from a white cell called 'B lymphocyte'. This kind of immunity, which is useful in the confrontation with invaders, is connected with another sort of immunity which involves the 'T lymphocytes'. While antibodies might be compared to *bullets*, T lymphocytes are more like *soldiers*. Lymphocytes are specialized. T-killers undertake *reconnaissance* and the selective destruction of specific *targets*. There are also T-helpers – which help B lymphocytes to secrete antibodies – and T-suppressors – which moderate the secretion of antibodies. Depending on the ratio between these two kinds of T cells, the production of antibodies of the B cells is either stimulated or suppressed.

This army is able to renew itself continually. In just a matter of minutes, millions of new lymphocytes and billions of new antibodies are produced. Lymphocytes are made from specialized cells in the bone marrow, which is like a sort of *basic training ground*. The lymphocytes move on to the thymus (see Glossary, pp. 164–5) which is more like a *specialized training camp*. It is here that the lymphocytes realize their particular competence, and it is from the thymus that they get their name – 'T' lymphocytes. The thymus is a small gland situated immediately behind the top of the chest bone. For a long time it was known only to gastronomes. It is 'sweetbreads'. Its physiological function has always been mysterious. Relatively large at birth, its size increases during childhood, then gets much smaller after puberty. In old people it is a vestige of its former self. Only in recent years has the thymus been considered to be an essential organ in the immune system. Of course, other organs, such as the lymphatic nodes, also play an important role in immunity.

Even though the immune system is dispersed, nevertheless it has a unity within it. It is like a national defence which coordinates the action of all the armed forces. Apart from combating bacteria, the immune system is at war with invaders as diverse as viruses, parasites, fungus spores or cancer cells. Of course, the immune system can make mistakes; it can hit the wrong target, or even turn the guns on itself in which case the antibodies destroy the cells they should be protecting. That is what is meant by 'auto-immune disease'. The immune system can also overreact to foreigners who are not really dangerous. This is what is meant by allergy. The immune system uses only a small part of the energy it has at its disposal. Put another way, the budget of the immune defences is small compared, for example, with the budget of the motor muscles.

Immunologists have to be convinced of the truth that life is a struggle and that struggling is a need. The immune system learns how to fight by fighting. But if the immune system does not get the chance to fight off certain viruses which usually attack in childhood, then it is a much more

21

difficult and exhausting battle as an adult. So it is better to get mumps at the age of four, rather than thirty-four.

## Barriers Which Get In The Way

The easiest barrier to smash between the various parts of the primal adaptive system is the one placed between the primal brain and the hormonal system. The hypothalamus belongs to the brain. It is made of nerve cells which communicate with other nerve cells by direct contact with their extended fibres. But the hypothalamus also belongs to the hormonal system. It secretes hormones on its own. These hormones reach the pituitary gland through the bloodstream. The hormones from the hypothalamus can either stimulate or inhibit the release of pituitary secretions.

The pituitary hormones in turn stimulate other endocrine

A feedback mechanism, showing the relationship between the hypothalamus, pituitary gland and adrenal gland

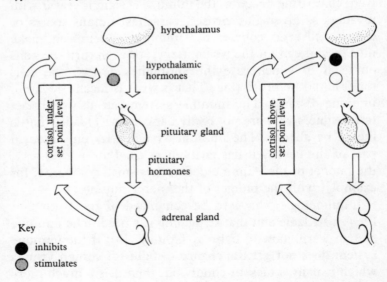

hypothalamus

hypothalamic hormones

cortisol under set point level

pituitary gland

pituitary hormones

cortisol above set point level

adrenal gland

Key

● inhibits

◯ stimulates

glands such as the adrenal glands, thyroid, ovaries and testicles. All these hormonal secretions (in the diagram cortisol is used as the model, but oestrogen, progesterone, and testosterone are other examples) control the activity of the hypothalamus by means of a feedback mechanism. Thus there is a real interdependence between the endocrine glands and the brain. What is more, the brain itself can now be considered as a gland with two exit doors; one which gives orders to the muscles and internal organs of the body through the nerve cells, and the other which gives orders to the whole organism through the hypothalamic hormones.

The brain can use the hormonal route, that is to say, chemical messengers, to send information from one part of itself to another. Nerve cells do not need to touch each other to communicate. For example, thirst can be triggered by injecting a small amount of a hormone called angiotensin into a precise zone of the brain; maternal behaviour can be induced in the same way by injecting some pituitary oxytocin. This phenomenon helps us to understand how small brain grafts can compensate for certain deficits. Physiologists and doctors who have a mental picture of cell-to-cell transmission, like an electronic network, might find it difficult to acknowledge the existence of certain substances which can modify the activity of the brain by a mechanism which is similar to the tuning of an orchestra.

A tougher barrier to smash is that which traditionally divides the hormonal system from the immune system. A few examples are enough to show that they are both part of a whole. Cortisol, the hormone secreted by the adrenal gland in situations of helplessness and hopelessness, depresses the immune system. It reduces the size of the thymus. It reduces the number and inhibits the activity of the T cells. It inhibits the synthesis of proteins in general and of antibodies in particular. In fact, the thymus itself is an endocrine gland which can secrete different kinds of

23

thymosine. These thymosines take part in controlling the secretion of different kinds of stress hormones by the feed-back mechanism.

It is not only cortisol which plays a role in all immune reactions. All the stress hormones do. Noradrenalin binds itself to surface receptors of lymphocytes and of other white cells and normally inhibits their function. Endorphins, which are natural pain-killers secreted by the primal brain, also influence the activity of the immune system.

In fact, every kind of hormonal secretion plays a role in immunity – not just the stress hormones. For example, the growth hormone is needed to maintain or restore the functions of T lymphocytes. The fusion between the hormonal system and the immune system is even more obvious since we know that lymphocytes themselves can produce ACTH, the hormone which stimulates the adrenal gland, and can also produce endorphins. We also know that lymphocytes have surface receptors for a wide variety of hormones. Of course, there are still many questions to which we don't yet know the answers. Even so, any kind of distinction between the hormonal system and the immune system can now be said to be obsolete.

What is perhaps even more difficult for many scientists and doctors is to fuse together their mental pictures of the primal brain and the immune system. For that reason it may be helpful to mention some research findings, some old, some new.

For many years it has been well known that there are nerve endings in the different organs of the immune system (thymus, bone marrow, spleen, lymphatic nodes). Certain lesions and certain stimuli of nerves are also known to have important effects on the number and activity of cells in these organs. Also, we now know that stimulating the immune system sends a flow of information to the hypo-thalamus. Some antigens – that is substances which stimu-late the immune system – can considerably increase the electrical activity of certain nerve cells of the hypothalamus. So the immune system can now be seen as an actual sensory organ which gives information to the brain.

Some spectacular experiments on the conditioning of immune reactions allow us to predict that the marriage between the nervous system and the immune system will be a thrilling new topic. Such a theoretical breakthrough might have enormous practical consequences. The American scientist Ader did an experiment on animals using taste aversion. He gave them saccharinated water at the same time as injections of a drug which depressed the immune system and which triggered digestive troubles. He then found that he could depress the immune system of these animals by giving them saccharinated water alone. Although Pavlov had already foreseen the possibility of conditioning the immune system, and although Metalnikov had shown during the 1920s at the Pasteur Institute in Paris that conditioning can change the response of an organism to an infectious agent, no one would have attempted to talk about educating the immune system even fifteen years ago.

Modern science is able to point not only to the unity of the primal adaptive system, but also to the incessant circulation of information inside this infinitely complex network. Modern science considers this circulation of information as a form of energy. Indeed, the primal adaptive system has a lot in common with traditional Oriental theories about the circulation of energy.

Just as traditional Oriental medicine thinks of disease as a disturbance of the channels of energy, so we can interpret disease as a disturbance of the primal adaptive system. After a great many detours, Western science will soon discover that Eastern traditions have passed on a profound understanding of human beings and of health.

Eastern traditions also understood the importance of fetal life and infancy. They knew this period formed the foundation on which the rest of a person's life was built. In ancient China, they used to practise 'embryonic education' (Tai-Kyo), the basic principle of which is that only a happy and healthy mother can have a happy and healthy baby. There are many proverbs inspired by the teachings of Tai-Kyo. For example; 'If you want to know a person, look at his mother.' In the *Caraka Samhita,* an Indian tradition, the development of the embryo and the fetus is studied during the third and fourth week of pregnancy, then month by month up to the seventh month. There are long chapters about fertility, conception, pregnancy and the newborn baby. In the Tibetan tradition *r Gyud-b Shi* the fetus is studied week by week.

## Early Development of the Primal Adaptive System

Thanks to recent scientific research, it is now possible for us to see the primal adaptive system as one whole. We also know that this system develops and reaches maturity during the time of close dependence on the mother.

When modern science talks about 'the archaic brain' or 'the primitive structures of the brain' it means the oldest part of the brain, both in the history of life and in the history of each human being. The primal brain is roughly the same among all mammals, from the most primitive right up to man. The primal brain reaches its maturity very early in the life of a human being, in the period of fetal life, birth and infancy. So the information going to the brain during this crucial period affects the course of some very important stages of its development.

The hypothalamus receives important information directly from the sensory organs and also from receptors which are sensitive to temperature and to the composition of the blood. Eastern traditions knew that by stimulating the senses, energy was brought to the brain. Western science is now able to prove that this is so. It is as if the brain needs to be recharged like a battery. For example, when the retina receives light, it transforms the vibratory energy of the light into electric energy at the optic nerve, then into chemical energy at the synapses between two nerve cells. When you stroke a baby's skin it gives energy to the brain at an important stage in its development.

A lack of sensory stimulation during the primal period could have far-reaching consequences. For example, when a pregnant woman is advised to spend a long time resting in bed, it is possible that the baby might lack sensory stimulation. In other words, there is a lack of energy transmitted to the brain at a stage when the primal brain is not yet mature. During life in the womb, the part of the inner ear which gives information about the body's movements and which will later on give a sense of balance (the vestibular system) reaches maturity very early on. The vestibular system of the fetus is constantly being stimulated when the mother is walking, dancing, changing her position, and so on.

There is recent evidence that the lateral part of the hypothalamus contains specialized cells which can transform some sensory stimulation into a feeling of pleasure. The period when the primal brain is reaching maturity might be the period when the hedonic capacity – the capacity to feel pleasure – develops. Modern science can now show us that the environment plays a role in the way the hypothalamus adjusts itself and reaches its appropriate levels at the beginning of life.

The way in which the brain becomes masculine or feminine is also becoming better understood. The permanent effects of sex hormones on the brain during the period surrounding birth are now accepted. This is a critical period which determines the sexual behaviour of the adult. For example, genetically male animals who had a temporary lack of male hormones during this short but critical period will, as adults, be sexually excited by the postures of

27

animals of the same sex, even if their level of male hormones is normal at that time.

In general, the entire hormonal profile is regulated during the primal period. The different parts of the primal adaptive system reach their maturity in a synchronized way. The hormonal system matures very early. At an early stage of fetal life the pituitary gland, which controls all the other endocrine glands, can secrete all the known pituitary hormones. None of these hormones is specifically to do with fetal life; the pituitary hormones of the fetus have exactly the same targets as an adult's and trigger exactly the same responses. What makes the hormonal system of the fetus special, however, is that it develops in an environment which is rich in placental hormones, and to a lesser degree, maternal hormones. When the fetus is eleven and a half weeks old, the vessels that will become the hypothalamus and pituitary glands come together. By that time the hypothalamus is already controlling the pituitary gland. And by the time the fetus is three months old, the day-to-day variations in the stress hormone ACTH are already well established.

There is a general rule which says that the history of an individual (ontogenesis) follows the pattern of the history of life (phylogenesis). Thus, however we look at it, our immune system is very archaic indeed. Phagocytes, a type of white blood cell which engulfs and swallows up foreign bodies, are as old as the oldest single-celled thing, protozoa. Lymphoid tissue, thymus, spleen and antibodies are all as old as the oldest vertebrates; the immune system in all the mammals is roughly the same as in man. During life in the womb, the order in which the different parts of the immune system develop has exact parallels with the history of life as a whole. The lymphoid cells and the thymus appear as early as the eighth week. Thanks to these tissues, the fetus can already produce high-weight antibodies (IgM) in case a bacterial disease is transmitted by the mother. Normally at birth the baby has only low-weight antibodies (IgG) which crossed the placenta. From birth, the baby's immune system must be stimulated. There follows a critical period during which time the IgM reach their definitive level, at about nine months of age. During this period, the baby is protected against the infections his mother had in the past, thanks to the low-weight antibodies which crossed the placenta. The baby is also protected by special antibodies called IgA and by various anti-infectious substances in the colostrum and milk. The composition of the mother's milk helps in the development of 'lactobacillus' in the baby's intestines which defends against the multiplication of dangerous bacteria. A good balance of bacteria in the intestines is needed to stimulate the intestinal lymphoid system and the local production of antibodies (IgA).

It is important to remember that the different parts of the primal adaptive system develop simultaneously and reach their maturity during the period of dependence on the mother. This simultaneous development is yet another argument pointing to the unity of this system.

Of course, this system has a constant exchange with the environment; it is not a 'closed' system. Communication with the exterior environment is made by eating, breathing and sensory stimulation. The primal adaptive system also has at its disposal that infinitely complex data bank, that extraordinary supercomputer – the neocortex, the 'associative brain'. This new brain reaches maturity very late both in the history of life and in the life of an individual. It continues to develop late into adulthood. Its enormous potential is the essential characteristic of man. It receives information from the outside environment through the sensory organs, and from the whole body through specialized receptors. It is through the neocortex that we know about the world of time and space and can communicate through language in such a sophisticated way. However, in adult humans the neocortex is so highly developed that it tends to overcontrol and repress the activity of the primal brain. Indeed, it can do this to such an extent that it inhibits those physiological functions which are most vulnerable, such as childbirth and the sexual act.

But however much the neocortex assumes control, the primal brain will still be primal in the sense of being first in importance. It is the primal brain which gives us the urge to survive as an individual and through procreation. It is also the primal brain which gives us a sense of belonging to the universe, a religious sense, a spiritual dimension. The neocortex may be considered to be the seat of the rational; the primal brain the seat of the irrational. The struggle for life is itself irrational. Thus the neocortex can be seen as a tool to be used in every aspect of the struggle for life, and in the survival of the individual, the group or the species.

The primal brain – the emotional brain – can also communicate with the emotional brain of other humans, and of animals. Empathy, sympathy, antipathy, attachment, love and hate are all to do with this kind of communication. Subtle ways of communicating such as this still have a mystery about them.

This new concept of the primal adaptive system can only be assimilated slowly and with difficulty, especially in the case of doctors and scientists. It will have to wipe out some indelibly printed pictures. During a recent discussion on French television a singer claimed that singing has effects on the immune system. This provoked a well-known medical journal to make fun of such a claim. Which only goes to show that it is more difficult for a doctor to wipe out the imagery associated with the word health than it is for a singer.

# CHAPTER 3

# Le Terrain*

Human beings have always dreamed of a bygone golden age, a paradise lost, a world without guilt and disease. The dominant medical ideology of the West is permeated by this myth. Doctors always look for the cause of each disease, and for each disease they look for the appropriate treatment. When Louis Pasteur said that micro-organisms could be a causative factor in infectious diseases his ideas won immediate acceptance. Since Pasteur there has been a succession of acclaimed victories in many fields.

Tobacco for example, has been found to be a causative factor in lung cancer; too much animal fat in the diet is a causative factor in cardiovascular diseases. Many viruses have been discovered and the part they play in many diseases understood. The recent discovery of the Epstein-Barr virus is often quoted as one of these victories. This virus has been found to be a causative factor in infectious mononucleosis, or glandular fever, a benign disease which is common in the Western world, and cancer of the lymphoid tissue, which is common amongst some Africans. Still more recently, a short time after AIDS became known

* See Linguistic note, p. 8.

31

as a specific disease, it was considered a victory to have isolated the causative virus, HTLV3. Indeed, there are countless such victories!

## Unanswered Questions

On the other hand, when you put the question another way round and ask what constitutes good health, medicine has far less to say. Perhaps this is to hide a lack of knowledge. One question which might be asked, for example, is why did two-thirds of humanity escape the plague during the fourteenth century? Another might be why do 90 per cent of the adult population of the Western countries have antibodies against the Epstein-Barr virus when they have never had any apparent disease? Another question might be why do only a minority of people infected by the HTLV3 virus develop AIDS? Why can some women give birth to their first baby in a few hours without any medical help? To ask questions like these is to ask about what I am calling *le terrain*. Even during Pasteur's time, there were men such as Antoine Béchamp (see Historical note, pp. 154–7) who thought about such questions, even if they did not actually use the word *terrain* in this context.

It was probably in Algeria that I first became aware of the concept of *terrain*. During the Algerian War, I was practising both military and civilian surgery there. Wounded people from both sides used to come to the hospital; some were Europeans, others were Berbers (Kabyles). When they came in with abdominal injuries we knew that the prognosis was better for the Berbers than for the Europeans with similar wounds. It was the same story with the civilian cases. Berbers with peritonitis were admitted at a very late stage of the condition. Even so, they healed incredibly easily. The local surgeon told me the Berbers had bellies of iron – they could withstand just about anything! At that time I was young enough to be influenced by what I saw and to have my own medical preconceptions swept away.

Some recent findings might throw some light on what *terrain* is all about. It is well known that Eskimos eat a lot of fish, so they assimilate a lot of a particular kind of unsaturated fatty acids. It is also well known that Eskimos are at low risk of heart disease, and to some extent cancer. It is tempting to make a connection between these two facts as Eskimo blood has a low concentration of a certain fatty acid which plays an essential part in thrombosis. But, however, things got more complicated when it was found that when Eskimos ate a Western diet, their level of this fatty acid still remained low. In fact, the way Eskimos metabolize food is different. It is as if their biological computers were programmed in another way.

It is observations like this which make us ask about the notion of *terrain* and also about the genesis of good health. But this kind of question is always dodged in our society. The priorities are directed much more to fighting each illness as it comes along. So, up against the notion of *terrain*, doctors seek easy refuge by talking about 'genetic factors'. But in fact the twentieth century is an extraordinary laboratory which has demonstrated to us that we should not overestimate the importance of genetic factors. The *terrain* which characterizes a particular individual was not cast in concrete the day when an egg and a sperm met. In our century, extraordinary movements of population have been made possible. People from every continent and every ethnic group have been thrown together and for several generations have shared the same lifestyle, including during the primal period of life – the time in the womb, birth and the period of infant feeding. In this century, the tendency has been for everyone to have a standardized state of health and disease.

Today one can claim that *le terrain* is an intricate mixture of hereditary and genetic factors and the way our biological computers were programmed at the time of dependence on the mother. But in order to evaluate these two components of *terrain*, we should first take a look at this rising new field of genetics to see what it knows about the origin of disease.

## Genetic Factors

It is well known that some diseases are hereditary; they are entirely determined by chromosomes from the father's sperm or from the mother's egg. Some hereditary diseases had been identified, of course, long before genetics emerged as a field of scientific study. In the *Talmud*, for example, circumcision was not advised in Jewish families where a member suffered from uncontrollable bleeding. As early as the beginning of the nineteenth century the rules of how haemophilia was transmitted were well known. About a thousand diseases can certainly be considered to be genetic. Some of them affect both men and women and there is a fifty-fifty chance of the disease being passed on to the children. The most common disease of this type – and probably the commonest genetic disease – is otosclerosis, a progressive deafness which starts in adulthood. It affects about one in a thousand. A second type of genetic disease, also affecting both men and women, is passed on by the specific chromosome from both parents, who are usually only carriers of the disease and do not suffer from it. The most common disease of this type is cystic fibrosis, which affects about one in every two thousand. The symptoms include severe digestive disorders, difficulty with breathing and lung infections. The third type of genetic disease is sex-linked. The best known is haemophilia, which does not affect girls at all. But the most common is probably Duchenne dystrophy, which only affects boys but is transmitted by females. It affects one child in every five thou-

34

sand and the main symptom is a progressive weakness of the muscles.

Diseases which are determined entirely by chromosomes are very rare. But there is much more to be learned from the field of genetics than from diseases which are purely genetic in origin. The field of genetics has also discovered a great deal about predisposition to particular diseases. For example, it has been shown that people with blood group A have a statistically higher chance of getting stomach cancer than those with blood group O, who are more likely to get duodenal ulcer. Similarly, the relationship between tissue typing (HLA) and certain diseases is becoming better known all the time. For example 90 per cent of insulin-dependent diabetics have DR3 or DR4 HLA antigens, while only 55 per cent of the population has these tissue types.

Above all, however, genetics has now entered a new era with the discovery of the polymorphism of DNA. DNA deserves a special mention. To be interested in biology these days without understanding the role of DNA is like trying to understand the word health without knowing what the hypothalamus is. DNA is the key to life. DNA is a unique molecule. It is the only thing which can make perfect copies of itself. It is why living matter is able to make living matter. Within DNA is the genetic code. We now know that there are marked differences between one person's DNA and another's. Thanks to our knowledge about the polymorphism of DNA, it is theoretically possible to predict which diseases healthy people are susceptible to. Such technical breakthroughs might give the institution of medicine, particularly genetics, a bigger and bigger role in our society. One can imagine a comeback of folk such as the famous French theatrical character Doctor Knock who said, 'Every healthy person has an illness he doesn't know about.' This was the quickest way to make the whole community ill.

# Primal Health

We learned nothing in the past from the countless and endless discussions on the respective roles of genetics and environment in the origin of certain diseases. The volume of articles and books attempting to evaluate the part of genetics in depression, obesity, schizophrenia or high blood pressure, for example, is often in direct proportion to the volume of our ignorance. The debates have always been passionate.

There are some kinds of people who have a tendency always to minimize the role of genetic factors. This is common among psychologists, whatever school they belong to. The behavioural psychologists, who emphasize a stimulus-response mechanism, have a tendency to explore the external world, rather than look inside the organism. Psychoanalysts, on the other hand, tend to emphasize the importance of childhood experiences. I know some psychoanalysts who will frown and change the subject when you dare to hint at genetics.

Other people, on the contrary, stress the importance of genetic factors. They feel relieved, even triumphant, when the genetic factors in some diseases are brought to light. This approach is common among doctors and scientists who are more comfortable with 'hard data', data which can easily be measured and written up in quantitative language. Hard data is often considered as the way to be respectable in conventional medical circles. However, this approach could be dangerous. When genetic factors are overestimated or overstressed, it means that environmental factors are ignored. This provides a good excuse for some practices, such as separating a newborn baby from its mother. It opens the door to an aggressive type of medicine, whose goal is to replace physiological processes. And it excludes another type of medicine – I call it nurturing medicine –

whose first aim is to satisfy basic needs without disturbing the physiological processes.

That is why, instead of concentrating on the part of genetic factors, we urgently need to be concerned with the other component of *terrain* – primal health. It is also why the genesis of good health should become a collective preoccupation. It is more constructive to be concerned with the way health is given a firm foundation in the fetus and baby than to know the names of all the illnesses to which your DNA predisposes you.

To evaluate primal health is not easy. Everyone who has tried to compare babies from different cultures, for example, has always been much more interested in their neuropsychic development or their psycho-motor development than in the state of their immune system or hormonal system. But it is likely that there are certain things in common with all these aspects of a baby's development, so such studies deserve to be considered. For example, when the anthropologist Marcelle Geber went to Kenya and Uganda to study the effects of malnutrition on newborn babies and infants, she was astounded to find that these babies were more advanced and smiled more than babies she had seen before in industrialized countries.

She found that around the age of six or seven months the Ugandan baby was able to pick up a toy which was outside its vision. With American and European babies, this is usually possible only at around fifteen months of age. Her test evaluated motor development, and the development of a form of reasoning. One big difference between the two groups was that the Ugandan babies belonged to a culture in which the period of dependence on the mother is not disturbed. Of course, the very different conditions of life make any comparison between the two groups difficult when it comes to things such as resistance to infection and allergies, and to changes in temperature and to lack of food. Even so, such cross-cultural studies can be useful preliminaries to a better understanding of the genesis of good health. The day when the genesis of good health is a priority, the risk of medical totalitarianism will be lessened. Good health is not the exclusive domain of one profession or of one institution, as the prevention of disease so often is.

# CHAPTER 4

# The Disease of Civilization

Depression, alcoholism, cardiovascular diseases, schizo-phrenia, obesity, rheumatism, allergies, auto-immune diseases, viral diseases, cancers – these are the words you hear most frequently when you talk about the diseases of civilization. Usually, the only reason why such apparently disparate diseases are ever listed together is because they are common in Western society. But, in fact, we now have good reason to think that this apparent diversity hides a common link between them all. All these diseases can be considered as the symptom of a weakness or disturbance of the primal adaptive system. Depending on genetic factors, on events which disturb the primal adaptive system at different stages of its maturation and depending on different triggering factors, the disease will take on different aspects. This is not very far from the Eastern theories which say that disease occurs either because of a weakness in the channels of energy or because of a disruption in the circulation of energy.

39

# A Unity Between Diseases

Modern science is now able to point out physiological disturbances and metabolic difficulties which most diseases of civilization have in common. It can now make connections – connections which were unimaginable even ten years ago – between diseases which medical specialization used to place poles apart. It is also now beginning to see how ignoring needs during the primal period could prepare the ground for the most common metabolic disturbances. Clearly, our society ignores fundamental needs which a human being has in its primal period – fetal life, the period around birth and infancy. Generally speaking, the existence of human needs which are fundamental, universal, cross-cultural and inscribed in our genetic code make it possible for us to determine the limits of human adaptability. The rediscovery of needs which are fundamental to humans will become an essential task for our industrialized society.

Take, for example, a newborn baby who is not allowed to sleep with its mother. Such indeed is the fate of millions of human beings in the Western world. Let us see how this might have long-term consequences. You do not need exceptional powers of observation to discover that all newborn babies need close contact with their mothers, particularly at night, in the dark. If this innate need, this primal need for close contact with an always available mother is not met, then the baby will demand and cry to start off with. But his cries may not bring his mother's arms. Instead, she is likely to switch on the light and give him something to eat. All too soon the baby loses all hope of being helped during the night, a time when he has a real need to be cuddled.

This particular situation comes under the heading of what physiologists call 'hopelessness' and 'helplessness' or 'inhibition of action'. All such situations carry with them a tendency towards reduced activity, sadness and indifference. One can only call it a tendency because this is not a catastrophic situation and many babies will have enough rewards during the day to compensate for privations during the night. Even so, these nightly experiences of helplessness are likely to leave their mark. And because it is happening on a widespread scale it deserves our attention all the more.

Situations such as these create a specific hormonal state at an age when the basic adaptive system has not yet reached maturity. The stress hormones have to adapt to this situation. In particular the level of cortisol secreted by the adrenal gland is high and the level of melatonin secreted by the pineal gland is low. The level of cortisol is high whenever there is any kind of inhibition of action. As for melatonin, it needs darkness to be secreted by the pineal gland. Cortisol and melatonin have a multitude of targets. These hormones play a role in most of the main metabolic pathways; in other words the chemical factories in our bodies where substances are made from the food we eat. It is particularly their action on the metabolism of unsaturated fatty acids on which we will concentrate now.

This takes us to an important crossroad – how prostaglandins are made. This crossroad is a key, and helps us understand how there can be a unity between various pathological conditions which on the face of it do not seem to have anything in common.

Prostaglandins have been well known since the Nobel Prize was awarded in 1982 to scientists working in this field. Like hypothalamus, T lymphocytes and DNA, prostaglandins is a word not to be ignored, even if you are not a scientist. Prostaglandins are local regulators of cell activity. They have a very short life indeed, working on a second-to-second basis. They are just about everywhere, in every cell and body tissue. Prostaglandins are classified as belonging to series 1, 2 or 3, depending on which family of fatty acid they are derived from. At this point it is impossible to study in detail all the possible effects of all

41

the known prostaglandins; the subject is too new and too complex. Nevertheless, we can see how extraordinarily diverse their actions are by taking as an example what we know about prostaglandins series 1.

Prostaglandins 1 are able to dilate the small blood vessels, thus lowering blood pressure. They inhibit the proliferation of cells of the smooth muscles which are in the vessel walls, so having an action on their calibre. Prostaglandins 1 inhibit the aggregation of a type of white blood cell called platelets; when the platelets bunch up together and clog the blood vessels there is a risk of thrombosis. They inhibit the synthesis of cholesterol, and help to halt the inflammatory process. They play an important role in the thymus, and their action on the maturation of T lymphocytes is comparable to that of thymic hormones.

It is not hard to imagine therefore that problems with the synthesis of prostaglandins 1 can have several consequences. In fact, this is what is happening to the newborn baby who is separated from its mother; the high level of cortisol blocks the synthesis of prostaglandins, particularly series 1, and the low level of melatonin cannot compensate for this. It is precisely this imbalance between the different prostaglandins which characterizes most of the diseases of civilization. Usually the synthesis of prostaglandins 1 is too low and the synthesis of prostaglandins 2 tends to be relatively high. Prostaglandins 2 exaggerate the inflammatory process when their synthesis and action is not modulated by prostaglandins 1. When you know how pervasive prostaglandins are you can see how an imbalance between them can be responsible for a wide range of disparate symptoms. What we know about prostaglandins reveals the uniformity behind the apparent plurality masking the diseases of civilization. A review of the main aspects of *the* disease of civilization will throw light on some hidden facts.

# Depression

Depression can be considered as the prototype of *the* disease of civilization. The number of depressed people in the world can be counted in hundreds of millions. It affects all ages and all social classes. The symptoms of depression are well known: sadness, the loss of the will to live and the struggle to survive and apathy. Physiologists know how to create experimental depression. It is easy – all they have to do is separate the newborn baby animal from its mother.

The hormonal disturbances which go with depression are now better understood. Indeed, much has been written about the depletion of hormones such as noradrenalin and serotonin in depression. But it is the high level of cortisol, and the consequent low level of prostaglandin series 1 which links depression to other aspects of *the* disease of civilization. This rise in the level of cortisol has a greater or lesser effect depending on the person's age. In a baby or young child a raised level of cortisol has a spectacular effect in reducing the size of the thymus. This organ is big only in babies and children, when the thymus is at its most active. The thymus is set to have a limited number of cell divisions during a lifetime. A high level of cortisol in babies has the effect of accelerating the ageing process of the thymus, and thus of the individual.

Some aspects of depression seem to be more and more common, perhaps because they are becoming better known. Seasonal depression is one of these. The symptoms of seasonal depression start in autumn and last up to the end of winter. It seems that patients with seasonal depression are not properly adapted to darkness, and that light might be the best treatment. It is likely that a disregulation of the pineal gland plays a role in this type of depression.

Regardless of age or of the function of the pineal gland,

43

however, a high level of cortisol disturbs the synthesis of prostaglandins.

## Alcoholism

When your level of prostaglandins 1 is rather low, you feel unhappy. The chances are that you will then search for a drug to boost your spirits – alcohol. A small amount of alcohol boosts the level of prostaglandins 1. It makes you feel better straightaway. The trouble is that the release of prostaglandins can only take place by depleting the stock of a particular fatty acid, which is the precursor of prostaglandins 1. The name of this precursor deserves recognition. The fact that human breast milk is one of the only natural sources of this fatty acid suggests its paramount importance. Its name is gamma-linolenic acid – or GLA for short. An adult must be able to synthesize GLA, because there are almost no foods which contain it. GLA is synthesized from linoleic acid, found mainly in seeds and seed oils, like sunflower seed. Any deficit of GLA reduces the synthesis of prostaglandins and also upsets the balance between the different kinds of prostaglandins. Alcohol has the effect of depleting the stock of GLA, so the level of prostaglandins 1 drops. Because a little alcohol makes you feel good, there is a great temptation to drink a little more, then a little more. It is a vicious circle – that is alcoholism. Chronic alcoholics make the deficit of prostaglandins 1 even worse, and they are more at risk than other people of developing other aspects of *the* disease of civilization.

## Hypertension

Hypertension and heart disease are two of the most commonly-quoted diseases of civilization. The usual expla-

44

nations for the frequency of hypertension are the strains and stresses of our lifestyle. The overworked businessman immediately springs to mind. Modern life has made everything more complex, more competitive, more ruled by the clock. Added to that, we put forward what seem to be the plausible explanations of bad diet, lack of exercise and some hereditary factors. However, those who have attempted to compile a list of the most stressful situations in our society put losing a partner or a loved one at the top of that list. But losing a loved one is not something which is specific to our society. So the question is, are we losing our ability to adapt? Are our capacities lower than they used to be, so that we are now always stretching our capabilities to the limit?

No one ever asks how the hypertensive person adjusted his adaptive mechanisms at the beginning of his life. Yet this would be a fruitful question to explore. Not long ago a young psychologist spent some time in our maternity unit at Pithiviers and she became convinced of the long-term importance of a newborn baby's first experiences. Then she spent some time in a hospital unit specializing in hypertension. She recounted this experience to me and told me about the sort of patients she had met there and what kind of personalities they had. I asked her what she knew about how these patients had been fed as babies. Of course, she did not know anything about that. Because a question like this, if not absurd, was at least not the kind of question anyone had ever thought of asking in a modern hospital.

But the question is not so absurd. The important role played by the hypothalamus in regulating blood pressure has been demonstrated many times. For example, if one specific zone of the hypothalamus is stimulated, the blood pressure is raised; if another zone is stimulated, the blood pressure is lowered. So it is not difficult to understand that when a newborn baby is in situations which trigger the release of stress hormones, he is regulating his hypothalamus in such a way that the seeds for hypertension are sown.

Yet again, it is the high level of cortisol and the low level of prostaglandins 1 which brackets hypertension with other aspects of *the* disease of civilization. The lack of prostaglandins 1 involves many factors which can lead to hypertension and cardiovascular disorders in general: the constriction of the small vessels; the thickening of the vessel walls; a tendency to thrombosis; and a rise in the level of cholesterol. Studies have shown a strong correlation between a higher risk of coronary disease and a low concentration of the direct precursors of prostaglandins 1 in the fat tissues.

Hypertension is a good example of a disease of civilization, and it is truly artificial to separate it from the others. For example, hypertension is very common amongst alcoholics. A study was done which made a connection between these two aspects of *the* disease of civilization. It was pointed out that the absorption of alcohol is often intermittent. Each period when alcohol is not being absorbed is a kind of stress and the response to this stress is an increase in the secretion of those hormones which raise the blood pressure.

## Schizophrenia

It is known that a deficit of prostaglandins 1 has an effect on the nerve cells and on the speed of nervous conduction; so it would be reasonable to expect that such a deficit could lead to a wide variety of behavioural disorders. Indeed, there are some arguments to suggest that a deficit in prostaglandins 1 might be one of the keys to an understanding of the mental disease which is most representative of our society – schizophrenia.

A low level of prostaglandins 1 has been found in the platelets of schizophrenics. It is known that schizophrenia can go into remission after an epiletic fit or a fever, situations which increase the level of prostaglandins 1. Also, most of the drugs for schizophrenia stimulate the secretion of prolactin, a hormone which increases the level of prostaglandins 1. This does not contradict other theories. It is commonly accepted that schizophrenia might have something to do with too much dopamine, which is one of the brain's messengers. As there is an antagonism between prostaglandins 1 and dopamine, these theories are complementary. So it is now possible to make the claim that prostaglandins 1 play a role in the interaction between brain messengers, particularly dopamine and the endorphins. Similarly, theories which suggest a deficiency in the pineal gland are in no way contradictory; on the contrary. It is worth adding that a deficiency of prostaglandins 1 would explain the abnormalities in the immune system of some schizophrenics, and would support the theories suggesting the role of a virus.

## Obesity

Of all the diseases of civilization, obesity is perhaps the most difficult to study on its own. Like schizophrenia, it has attracted many speculative theories. Until recently it has been impossible to disassociate obesity from eating too much or having too big an appetite. But even with this simplistic view we are still led towards that centre of appetite, the hypothalamus, and the primal period of life when it is adjusting itself.

Some people are fat and some people are thin, even when they eat the same food. The discovery of brown fat is a clue to understanding why. Brown fat is situated chiefly behind the neck and in the back. One of the roles of brown fat is to burn up excess calories; it can do this thanks to some small energy-producing units called mitochondria.

The particular colour of brown fat comes from the large number of mitochondria. New research shows that some obese people have underactive brown fat, and their excess calories therefore turn into body fat. It seems that this faulty brown fat is accompanied by a lack of certain enzymes which can only work properly when there are enough prostaglandins 1. Much is still unknown; however, the genesis of obesity does indicate how artificial it is to put a solid barrier between obesity and other diseases of civilization.

## Rheumatism

Some kinds of rheumatism, conditions which involve excessive inflammatory reactions, seem to be a good example of an imbalance in the synthesis of different prostaglandins. People are often stricken with an acute attack of rheumatism a few months after an intense emotional upset; they are often exhausted and their level of cortisol is low, as if they had overstepped their capacity to adapt. The inflammation of rheumatism was first thought to be a result of an overproduction of prostaglandins 2, which are proinflammatory. But, in fact, what seems to be happening is that there is a lack of prostaglandins 1, which are antiinflammatory. When the level of prostaglandins 1 is artificially restored, the production of prostaglandins 2 goes down like a see-saw. This new way of looking at rheumatism might have enormous practical consequences.

Some forms of rheumatism are regarded as diseases of the immune system, and the role of some viruses has also been considered as possible. But, once again, this system of classifying diseases is obsolete.

# Depression of the Immune System

When a baby is faced with situations of helplessness and hopelessness at a stage when its immune system is being adjusted the consequences can be profound and can involve several mechanisms. Of course, there are elements involved in hormonal balance other than the high level of cortisol, and cortisol itself acts in many ways. For example, it inhibits the synthesis of proteins and thus the manufacture of antibodies.

If we consider the synthesis of prostaglandins as the starting point, we can then understand all the possible consequences when the function of the T lymphocytes is depressed. It is known that a lack of prostaglandins 1 acts as a block to the formation of the different T lymphocytes in the thymus. Generally speaking, T suppressors seem to be the most vulnerable to the action of cortisol and to a lack of prostaglandins 1. The role of the T suppressors is to control, to put the brake on the formation of some antibodies by the B cells. A lack of T suppressors is in fact what a number of diseases have in common, particularly allergies, where the reaction against certain foreign bodies is exaggerated.

# Allergies

In the last fifteen or so years there has been a spectacular increase in the frequency of allergic diseases, such as asthma, rhinitis, eczema and urticaria. A British study investigated the development of five thousand children born in 1946. It revealed that they had six times less chance of having eczema than their own children, and three times less chance of having asthma. It is also more and more difficult to define what an allergic illness is and the list gets longer and longer all the time.

Food allergies are also getting more common, although they are not yet well known because they are often hidden allergies. They are hard to detect because there may be a delay between the time when the food is eaten and the symptoms appear. The symptoms themselves seem to have little to do with food reactions and can often be taken for something else. They include depression, headaches, muscle or joint pains, palpitations and sweating. The foods in question are often those which are eaten everyday and which people sometimes like most. Before, the only way to detect these allergies was to put the individual on a fast and then introduce certain foods one by one. Now there are blood tests which can rapidly detect the reaction of the lymphocytes to different allergens.

Up to now, Western man was thought capable of adapting easily to a wide range of foods, but the growing intolerance to certain foods makes this questionable. The capacity to adapt has been shown by some groups of humans who could travel further and further from their place of origin in the tropics. The further north, the more people there are who have the advantage of being able to digest milk because they had the enzyme lactose. Is industrialized man now in the process of losing some of his capacities to adapt?

It would be easy to attribute this rise in the number of allergic diseases to the never-ending introduction of new allergens such as food additives or new industrial products. However, the causes are probably much deeper than this; from what we know now about allergies the first thing we should think of is the period of infant feeding.

Perhaps the best way of causing experimental allergies is to copy some habits which are widespread in the twentieth century. We could start by separating the baby from its mother in the hours following birth so that the baby does not take all the colostrum he could have done, had he stayed with his mother. It is known that colostrum, which precedes milk, contains antibodies IgA which line the intestine walls and make them less vulnerable to foreign proteins. Second, we could follow the practice of giving this newborn baby a little bottle of artificial milk, so he does not die of hunger, the poor thing. This one 'little' bottle, given to the baby before the mother's milk has come, at a stage when the baby's intestinal mucous membrane is at its most permeable, is exactly what will make the baby sensitive to foreign proteins.

When this baby is three or four months old, we could start mixed feeding. This means greatly increasing the number of antigens to which the baby might be sensitive at a stage when his immune system is immature. At this age, all the baby needs is his mother's milk. Introducing mixed feeding so early also has other disadvantages. Because the baby gets the calories he needs from solid foods, he demands less and less mother's milk and so takes in less and less GLA, that precious precursor of prostaglandins 1 which only human milk can give him in sufficient quantities. The last common habit we might adopt is to separate mother and baby during the night. This would have the effect of raising the level of cortisol in the baby and reducing the production of milk in the mother.

If we copy all these common habits we can be sure of multiplying the ways to disturb the maturation of T lymphocytes. We can also be sure of multiplying the number of allergic conditions.


## Auto-Immune Diseases

The lack of T suppressors, which are the most vulnerable when there is a low level of prostaglandins 1, is also the common link between all the auto-immune diseases.

An auto-immune disease is a bit like physiological suicide. It is as if someone starts to self-destruct when he

51

feels he is in some situation with no way out, that is, a situation of helplessness or hopelessness. Genetic factors often seem to be associated with auto-immune diseases. For example, people with the tissue type HLA-DR3 are known to be particularly susceptible to diabetes, some thyroid diseases and defects in the adrenal glands. It does not mean that people with this particular tissue type will get any of these diseases; neither does it mean that everyone who carries the particular antibodies will necessarily show the symptoms of these diseases. Other people with a different tissue type might, in the same emotional state of helplessness, make antibodies which attacked other organs, such as the muscles.

The cells of all the endocrine glands (except perhaps the pineal gland) can be targets of auto-immune reactions. This shows yet again that there is absolutely no division between diseases of the immune system and diseases of the endocrine system. However, the endocrine glands are not the only targets of auto-immune reactions. The target organ could be, for example, the digestive tract. Auto-immune diseases in this category are some types of gastritis, stomach and duodenal ulcers, and ulcerative colitis.

Not all auto-immune diseases restrict their attack to one organ only. Some have widespread effects on the body, such as rheumatoid arthritis or systemic lupus. The whole subject of auto-immune diseases is getting larger and more complicated every day. It may be that not all the auto-antibodies are destructive; some might act as stimulators. Among the diseases with stimulating auto-antibodies may be found certain conditions involving an overactive thyroid gland side by side with certain duodenal ulcers. In general, studies on auto-immune diseases, and also some family studies, show that there is a close relationship between disorders of the thyroid and disorders of the stomach. Such evidence which blurs the divisions between the different medical disciplines poses a huge challenge to specialized medicine as it is today.

## Viral Diseases

It is possible that a virus may be implicated in some auto-immune diseases such as diabetes and multiple sclerosis. The prostaglandins may again be a key. A lack of prostaglandins 1 blocks the maturation and function of T lymphocytes so that the resistance to viruses is lowered. When there is a viral infection, this can block the synthesis of prostaglandins 1 and so weaken the body's defence system in a vicious circle.

The younger a person is when he first meets a virus, the greater are his chances of controlling it and establishing a permanent immunity. When there is a lack of T suppressors, there is a higher risk of viral infections. So when you have an allergic disease, you have a lower resistance to viral infections. An example of this is a generalized reaction after a smallpox vaccination.

As time goes on, more of the frontiers between allergic diseases, auto-immune diseases and viral diseases are being destroyed. We might ask whether modern man is especially vulnerable to viruses? At the moment the common anxiety of mankind is about nuclear war. But does not the real danger for mankind perhaps lurk in a virus? The sudden development of viral diseases like AIDS or herpes might serve as a warning.

## Cancer

It is becoming better known that cancer can manifest itself after an emotional crisis, such as grief. Emotional states like this depress the immune system. The depression of the role of the T lymphocytes makes us question the origin and development of cancer. It is also well known that some viral diseases seem to set the scene for malignant tumours. At a molecular level, it is known that the cancerous cell lacks a particular enzyme which blocks the manufacture of the precious GLA. This means that the cancerous cell cannot synthesize prostaglandins 1. In laboratory experiments, it has been found that when GLA was added to malignant cells, these malignant cells were killed. (The scientists used cells from mice; some had melanoma, some cancer of the oesophagus, some had bone cancer and others had cancer of the liver.)

Some characteristics of cell cancers are well known nowadays, for example tumoral reversion. This means that under certain circumstances cancer cells can become normal again. We also know that, unlike other cells, they have lost what is known as contact inhibition, which means, for example, that cultures of cancer cells will go on multiplying even when they have completely colonized the bottom of a box. These phenomena suggest that the cancer cell is indifferent to hormonal orders. This indifference is apparently a consequence of changes in the cell membrane. This new knowledge about cancer cells is already diverting the attention of scientists towards those metabolic pathways which play such an important role in the constitution of cell membranes: the metabolic pathways of the fatty acids.

## Ageing

The different aspects of *the* disease of civilization can be interpreted as different ways to grow old. It would be simplistic to claim that it is only because curable diseases have been eliminated that we can now devote our attention to some pathological conditions which affect everyone, such as ageing.

It seems paradoxical to claim that early ageing is a characteristic of our society when the average life expectancy has never been so high as it is now. This statistically longer life is partly because technological medicine can now rescue people who would otherwise die, both old people and babies, and partly because the huge privations of former generations have now disappeared amongst populations with a high standard of living. This does not mean that we have learned how to delay ageing.

People who have tried to understand the process of ageing rarely pay any attention to the primal period of life when the baby is dependent on its mother and when its biological clocks are adjusting themselves. When situations beyond the baby's control depress its primal adaptive system, and when the size of its thymus is decreasing, a dent is made in the baby's stock of life. It is as if some capital is withdrawn from the deposit account of allotted years. Indeed, many facts confirm that longevity has a lot to do with the way the primal brain has been regulated. It is possible to prolong the life of rats by taking out the pituitary gland shortly after birth and compensating for this lack in adrenal hormones. Exercise also increases a rat's life, but only if it is begun at a very early age. Clinical studies suggest that the thinnest and fattest humans have the lowest life expectancy; these are the people whose biological computers were most maladjusted during the primal period of life.

We took the metabolism of unsaturated fatty acids and the synthesis of prostaglandins as a model of metabolic pathways which are commonly disturbed in our society. In fact, these metabolic difficulties cannot be disassociated from the ageing process. Indeed, the ageing process may be considered to be a blocking agent itself of the synthesis of unsaturated fatty acids. Certainly, early ageing can be considered as an aspect of *the* disease of civilization.

## Conclusion

This review of the most common pathological conditions in our society must not, of course, lead us to the conclusion that an imbalance between different series of prostaglandins is the only possible explanation. And there are probably many kinds of complex imbalances between different prostaglandins, even inside the same series, and especially inside the series 2. The common link between all the diseases must be seen more as a sign that the present divisions we have in medical specialisms have been made obsolete by new information. Once we get rid of those useless barriers medical disciplines have erected between systems of the body, a new era of medicine could open up where the prevention of diseases would become a discarded aim. The genesis of good health and the prevention of early ageing would then become more fruitful lines of research.

# CHAPTER 5

# Sexual Health

Health is not only the force which propels an individual to struggle for his own life; the dynamics of survival have other ways of expressing themselves. The need to procreate is one of them. The necessity of assuring the survival of the species expresses itself in sexual life and care given to children.

## Survival by Procreation

Survival by procreation needs several conditions. In the first place, there has to be attraction to and by an individual of the opposite sex. Second, behaviour and anatomy have to make the sexual act possible. Fertilization can only happen if the sexual cells – sperm and ova – develop until they are mature. Many conditions need to be fulfilled before the egg and the sperm can meet and fuse, including the composition of the sperm and of the cervical mucus and the action of the smooth muscles of the uterus and the fallopian tubes. Then, the uterus must be able to receive the egg. Third, the genes from the mother and father have to be compatible so that the new organism can survive.

57

The mother's body must be able to tolerate this graft in her womb, and provide favourable conditions so that the placenta and fetus can reach an ideal stage of maturity.

There must be no irreversible fetal distress during childbirth. Once the child is born, the conditions for procreation are still going on. These conditions include bonding between mother and baby, and general protective behaviour towards babies and infants from the adults around them. Breastfeeding is the last stage in the process of procreation.

When you list all these conditions and are aware of the incredible complexity of reproduction, you can see just how much the primal adaptive system is called upon in the course of sexual life. One can also see how various episodes in a person's sexual life can be very sensitive to weaknesses or disregulations of the primal adaptive system.

The mechanisms we have for survival by procreation are much more fragile than those needed for survival of an individual. According to the laws of biology, the survival of an individual is the priority. In the hierarchy of survival, sexual functions come lower down. When somebody's life is threatened, his sexual behaviour is depressed. So self-preservation can take priority over childbirth. When a female mammal is in labour, seeing a dangerous animal will frighten her and make her secrete hormones such as adrenalin. This will interrupt the blood supply to the uterus and placenta, and have the effect of sending blood rushing to the brain and muscles so that the animal can fight or run away quickly. But the price of survival for the mother could perhaps be a deadly fetal distress. It is through exactly the same mechanisms that any kind of fear will dramatically inhibit all aspects of a human's sexual life. In a society with such a multitude of ways to disturb fetal life, childbirth, the mother-infant relationship and breastfeeding, it is no wonder that there are problems at various stages of a person's sexual life.

Sexual problems are very wide-ranging in modern day society. A weak sexual appetite can be the main symptom of a mild depression. Depressed people are difficult to seduce, do not take the initiative, are not very sensual and have difficulty in reaching a state of sexual excitement. Other sexual difficulties have more to do with emotional immaturity. Some people have difficulties in forming any kind of attachment. But where does this capacity to form attachments, to make ties with other people, come from? In other words, where does the capacity to love come from?

## Attachment

It was only in the late 1950s that scientists began to ask and seek answers to such questions. It all started by observing the behaviour of animals. Most well known are the goslings studied by the German ethologist Konrad Lorenz. Lorenz observed that the goslings became attached for the rest of their lives to the first animal they had contact with after their birth. Indeed, some of the goslings continued to be attached to Lorenz himself all their lives. It was Lorenz who discovered the notion of 'sensitive period' – a critical period whose circumstances would never be repeated. Later on, other ethologists studied attachment in other birds and some mammals, particularly goats and primates.

Studies of the possible role of hormones in maternal behaviour began when Terckel and Rosenblatt injected the plasma from mother rats into either male or virgin rats. This had the effect of triggering maternal behaviour in the male and virgin rats. From studies such as this it became possible to demonstrate the role of different sex hormones, in particular the positive effects of oestrogen and prolactin. But some facts could not be explained by the action of these sex hormones alone. Other studies showed, for example, that this very same maternal behaviour could be triggered in the male and virgin rats when they were given prolonged contact with newborn animals. How could this be explained?

A new stage in this field of research was reached with the discovery of hormones from the brain and all the chemicals which come under the heading of endorphins, many of which seem to play a role in the bonding process.

But whatever scientific methods were used, the same conclusions were reached: there is a sensitive period, a critical period which leaves its imprint forever.

The first hour following birth might be one such sensitive period in humans. There is a great deal of evidence which makes us think this must be so. First and foremost, mothers witness this for themselves. During the hour following birth, the mother is in a very special state of consciousness where she is quite oblivious to everything going on around her – as long as nothing disturbs this first contact with her baby and nothing shatters this holy atmosphere. This is often the best time for the baby's first sucking.

Second, there are physiological reasons as to why the first hour after birth might be a sensitive period. The hormones which are secreted by both the mother and the baby during childbirth have not yet been eliminated during this first hour. They are basic to the process of attachment. In particular, mother and baby still have a high level of endorphins. When we know that opiates can create habits and dependent behaviour, and can also give rise to care-giving and affectionate behaviour, it is easy to understand why this first hour after birth can play such an important role in the process of attachment. A woman who has just given birth is in an especially vulnerable state. Knowing what we do about the process of attachment, it is not so hard to understand why she might easily form an attachment with somebody who is with her during that first hour after birth, such as a professional. It is not just by chance that traditional wisdom always excluded men from the place of birth.

The emotions we feel in everyday life involve various hormones, and it is these hormones which play a role in the process of attachment, particularly the endorphins. A mother and her newborn baby are awash with these endorphins just after the birth as long as nothing has been disturbed. This attachment between mother and baby is a vital episode in life, and is the model which is necessary for all other forms of attachment later on. During sexual intercourse partners are in close contact and at the same time have a high level of endorphins. All attachments, whether it is to humans, to animals, or to things, might not be very far from this first mother-baby model.

However, we must not run away with the idea that the process of attachment between mother and baby is just a rush of hormones at one short and sensitive period. Some people even suggest that the hormones involved in the process of attachment, such as ACTH and vasopressin as well as the endorphins, have already been secreted by the baby early in its fetal life so that the real attachment between mother and baby started well before birth.

The distance between the word attachment and the word love sums up the whole complexity of the human phenomenon. You can hardly talk about love using the language of physiology. The different vocabularies reflect the gulf between the animal and the human worlds. Of course, it will always be difficult to prove the importance of sensitive periods in humans because so many factors are involved, such as the culture to which a person belongs.

However, pioneers such as Marshall Klaus and John Kennell dared to attempt the study of sensitive periods in humans. They knew that the circumstances of the mother/baby relationship have as much of an effect on the

61

whole culture as the culture has on them. So when the early mother/baby relationship is either helped or hindered, it has consequences for the whole culture.

## Sexual Behaviour

The view outlined above of the process of attachment suggests a strong correlation between the early mother/baby relationship and the sexual life of the adult. It is hard to separate difficulties of attachment, emotional immaturity and the kind of sexual problems which therapists often encounter. These present themselves above all as difficulties in experiencing pleasure.

When you think of sex therapy, you think of male impotence, premature ejaculation, frigidity and all the problems to do with orgasmic insufficiency. But it would be possible to look at orgasmic insufficiency in a completely different way. The orgasmic state is characterized by a change in the conscious level which is a physiological regulator of the primal adaptive system.

Physiological changes in the level of consciousness have hardly been studied at all, except for sleep. Orgasm and birth have hardly been touched upon as areas for study from the standpoint of levels of consciousness. However, both have a strong impact on the primal adaptive system. The lack of interest from scientists in the physiology of orgasm and childbirth is in marked contrast to the great interest they have shown in artificially-induced states of consciousness, by drugs such as LSD or by techniques such as hypnosis or meditation.

There are, of course, many kinds of sexual behaviour which do not lead to the therapist's door. Such behaviour is deeply embedded in an individual's personality. There is a very wide spectrum between exclusively heterosexual and exclusively homosexual behaviour. Occasional homosexual behaviour, masculine or feminine, has been found in all civilizations, in every age of history and even among every kind of mammal, from mice up to apes. What seems to be special to our society now is the frequency of an exclusive or predominant homosexual behaviour among men. The origin of homosexuality is not yet fully understood, but when one begins to look into it more deeply one has to go back to the primal period of life.

It is now known that the sexual differentiation of the brain happens at the end of pregnancy or the period around birth. It is from this time that the brain becomes either masculine or feminine. Therefore, it follows that the sexual behaviour of adults might depend upon events which take place at this stage of development. The critical period for the sexual differentiation of the brain may vary slightly from one species to another, but it is always around the time of birth. It is thought that when the newborn opens its eyes this period of hormonal sensitivity is at an end.

What we know about the hormonal profile of homosexuals fits perfectly with the hypothesis of a transitory lack of testosterone during the critical period. Homosexuals usually have the same level of total testosterone as heterosexuals, but their level of testosterone which is not combined with other chemicals (free testosterone) is lower. The level of pituitary hormones which control testicular functions is relatively high and so is the level of oestrogens. The important thing to realize is that if this hormonal profile were to be artificially reproduced in an adult, it would not give rise to homosexual behaviour. When a fetus is faced with a lack of testosterone at the end of pregnancy it compensates for this by increasing secretions from the pituitary hormone. At the same time as the fetus increases the level of male hormones by a feedback mechanism it increases in parallel the level of oestrogens. In fact, oestrogen increases the binding capacity of sexual hormones with proteins so that the level of free testosterone is lower.

63

This raises the question: How and why do some fetuses lack male hormones at the end of pregnancy? The answer could be that certain stressful situations at this time might trigger a high level of activity in the mother's adrenal glands. The adrenal gland releases male hormones whose action is different from testosterone, but which are similar enough to be in competition with testosterone in the baby's brain. This produces what amounts to a lack of testosterone.

Since changes in the nervous and hormonal system go hand in hand with changes in the immune system at a time when all three systems have not yet reached maturity, it suggests that the immune system of homosexuals might have some peculiarities such as a specific susceptibility to some viruses which, in their turn, weaken the immune system.

When we consider the sexualization of the brain, we also have to consider how the brain reaches the rhythms which are appropriate to the particular sex and personality of the individual. It is now also known that hormonal secretions are cyclic and even pulsating. The generator of rhythm is situated in the primal brain, in precise zones of the hypothalamus.

The best known cycle is the female menstrual cycle. The secretion of sex hormones in women follows this rhythm; this is how it is possible for an egg to be released once a month. In our society, fertility problems connected with ovulation are common and often go with periods which are long, irregular or absent altogether. The best way to avoid such problems would be to make sure that the newborn girl is able to regulate the rhythm of her hypothalamus at the very beginning of her life. This would make her less vulnerable to future disturbances. The way to ensure this is to make sure the period of her dependence on the mother is not disturbed.

In fact, all hormonal secretions are pulsating and

rhythmic. It is now known that whole groups of nervous cells which secrete hormones go into action every hour or two to order the secretion of progesterone in women or testosterone in men. Every organ involved in reproduction shares this rhythmic activity. So the uterus seems to release prostaglandins in a pulsating sort of way in harmony with the rhythm of secreting pituitary oxytocin. Future generations will have mental pictures of the neuro-hormonal machine which will be very different from those we have had up to now. The concept of a brain which is constantly rhythmic and pulsating gives a new vision to what the ancients called 'vital energy'.

Every stage of reproduction puts the entire primal adaptive system to the test. Pregnancy might therefore be considered as a neuro-hormonal event and also an immune system event. How is the mother able to tolerate these grafts? First the egg and then the fetus and the placenta? This is still something of a mystery – although not a complete mystery because we know, for example, that progesterone which is secreted at a high level during pregnancy depresses the immune system. Sometimes, of course, this mysterious tolerance fails. It is likely that some fertility problems are due to an immunological reaction by the mother against her partner's sperm. Antibodies against sperm have been found in the blood and cervical mucus.

Some miscarriages might amount to graft rejection. Some conditions which affect the immune system, such as systemic lupus, make pregnancy difficult or even impossible. It is also known that some diseases of newborn babies are due to the action of maternal antibodies, for example certain kinds of jaundice where the mother's antibodies act against the baby's red blood cells, or purpura where the mother's antibodies act against the baby's platelets.

The shortcomings in compatability between mother and baby only serve to reinforce the biological mystery which still surrounds pregnancy and make us even more aware of the infinite complexity of the primal adaptive system. When you realize how little is known about this infinitely complex system, you have an even greater respect for physiology. What we should be doing is helping physiology, not disturbing it, not triggering a cascade of side-effects. Unfortunately, the institution of medicine has grabbed some episodes of sexual life for itself and has shown a marked tendency to play the role of the sorcerer's apprentice. This medical attitude is typified in the field of childbirth, a key event which has many far-reaching consequences.

## Childbirth

It could be said that the obsession to control characterizes the discipline of obstetrics. It has been like this ever since medical man entered the birthing room in the seventeenth century and created the basis of modern obstetrics. It was medical man who introduced the position of lying on the back; and it was medical man who founded midwifery schools. Midwives were no longer mothers helping other mothers, thanks to their personal experience and specifically feminine sensitivity. Instead, they became professionals who were taught how to control the birth process. Doctors were in competition with each other to control the training of midwives. As long as the Chemberlen family in the seventeenth and eighteenth centuries could keep the secret of their forceps and prove the superiority of their technique, it kept the monopoly on the training of midwives. This tendency to consider control as the priority became more pronounced as time went on. Now, in the era of electronics and ultrasound, the medicalization of childbirth is complete. It is becoming more and more obvious that one cannot control an episode of sexual life without disturbing it.

All over the world people are worried about the rise in the

number of caesarians and other obstetrical interventions. In the USA the caesarian rate has multiplied almost four times in the last fifteen years. More and more babies are born impregnated with drugs which had been given to the mother during childbirth. The number of babies who are separated from their mothers at birth and transferred to pediatric units has reached unbelievable proportions. Such practices should become a major concern for public health bodies.

In the search for answers it is easy to find explanations for the rise in the rate of caesarians. Fetal distress is now more easily and more frequently diagnosed than in the past; breech presentations more often lead to a caesarian; a caesarian is preferable to a difficult forceps delivery; when a woman has had a previous caesarian, a subsequent delivery by the vaginal route is rarely attempted. For the doctor, there are legal advantages in doing a caesarian; there are also financial advantages in some countries; recently there is the additional justification of genital herpes. Each of these explanations has some merit, but perhaps they hide what is essential.

What is essential to realize is that difficulties in childbirth come under the heading of diseases of civilization. In countries where they are reaching the third generation of medicalized birth, women are less and less able to give birth by themselves using their own hormones. Some of them lost this ability at the time of their own birth. By observing thousands of women and listening to what they had to say, I am convinced that there is a correlation between the way a baby girl is born and the way she will give birth to her own children. But, of course, things are not so simple, and we must not confuse correlation and similarity. One can never be certain beforehand whether a delivery will be easy or difficult. Nevertheless, when a woman knows that her mother brought her into the world herself, without drugs and without any medical intervention, she has the best

67

prognosis. These factors are more important than her age, the size of her pelvis and so on.

Knowing what we do about how important prostaglandins 1 and 2 are in the physiological process of childbirth, it is almost possible to make a prediction about an increase in difficulties during childbirth. An imbalance between these two prostaglandins is one of the main links between all the diseases of civilization. To stop this imbalance we must reconsider the basis of obstetrics. Our first goal should be to help women make the best use of their own physiological potential. We would have to openly recognize the real needs of a labouring woman. She needs intimacy; any interference of her privacy inhibits labour. But on the other hand she must not feel alone. An experienced and caring woman is often the only person who can satisfy all these apparently disparate needs. An authentic midwife is a mother helping other mothers give birth. By contrast, a masculine presence can block the labour. Warmth, semi-darkness, silence, whispered words – all these things reinforce intimacy and spontaneity and make it easier for the labouring woman to feel free to be in any position.

Childbirth is an extraordinary event for the primal adaptive system. During delivery it is the primal brain which regulates hormonal secretions. The best way not to disturb the activity of the archaic brain is to reduce the inhibitions which come from the new brain, from the neocortex. Above all, physiological childbirth is a change in the state of consciousness, a reduction in activity of the upper brain.

The hormones which play a role in childbirth are not only at work during this event, but are involved in every episode of sexual life. Whether we are talking about childbirth, intercourse or breastfeeding, we always find that the hormone adrenalin inhibits, whereas hormones like oxytocin and the endorphins positively encourage. Generally speaking, we can now make the claim that the capacity to feel pleasure and the capacity to cope with pain both bring into play the same physiological system. From modern physiology we can see that sexual life is a whole. One cannot go on creating massive disturbances in childbirth and breastfeeding without altering the sexual life and the capacity to love of society as a whole.

## Breastfeeding

The continuum of the physiological phenomena of pregnancy, childbirth and breastfeeding perfectly illustrates the unity of sexual life as well as the unity of the primal adaptive system. For example, during pregnancy the function of the T lymphocytes is depressed; perhaps because of the high level of hormones such as progesterone. This begins to explain how the mother can tolerate a gestating fetus, which is tantamount to a graft. During the critical period of childbirth the stress hormones such as catecholamines, cortisol and the endorphins tend to exaggerate this depression of the immune system. These hormones will already have prepared for what is to follow.

Certain endorphins make it easier for the hormone prolactin to be secreted, which completes the maturation of the baby's lungs. Afterwards, during the long period of breastfeeding, prolactin helps the mobilization of the fatty acid which is the precursor of prostaglandin 1. It is a way to get the T lymphocytes working again, and helps the immune system get back its former strength.

Giving the breast is in itself a form of preventive medicine. For a newborn baby the way it is fed may be considered a cornerstone of primal health. Unfortunately in our society, even if a woman feels the need and decides to breastfeed, she has to face a series of obstacles. The beginning of breastfeeding is often disturbed because the delivery itself was disturbed. Nowadays few women give birth using their own hormones. And in the context of our modern institutions many mothers and babies cannot have their need for complete intimacy and body contact satisfied during the first days following the birth. Having those basic needs met is the key to a good start in breastfeeding. Afterwards, modern woman, going back to the bosom of the nuclear family, has to obey other rhythms than those of her baby. The telephone, the ease of going from one place to another and going back to work are all sources of disturbance.

When something goes wrong with breastfeeding it is normal to call the doctor. But most doctors are not interested in that kind of thing and don't know what to do. So once you call a doctor it often means the end of breastfeeding. Breastfeeding counsellors who could give help from one mother to another are still very few in number. But, above all, many women have difficulties in breastfeeding because they were not breastfed well themselves. Experience shows that by taking the breast herself a baby girl begins to learn how to breastfeed her future children.

It is the same with childbirth. Women who give birth during the 1980s were themselves born at a time when formula feeding was in the ascendant; at a time when it was common to tell a mother not to give her baby bad habits, not to spoil him, to leave him to cry. They were also born into a male-dominated society where the model was masculine. Such a society does not give any glory to things which are the preserve of women and mothers.

Today, there is a new upsurge in breastfeeding, but whenever any difficulty arises there is a great temptation not to carry on. Formula milk is now said to be 'humanized', but this can lead to dangerous mistakes. No artificial milk will ever be able to replace mother's milk. Human breast milk may be considered as a living tissue containing millions of white blood cells which can kill bacteria;

enzymes which aid digestion; antibodies; and protective bacteria. Birth does not just mean arriving in the atmosphere, discovering gravity and joining human society. It also means meeting for the first time the world of bacteria. At birth the baby's digestive tract is sterile. In the next twenty-four hours, no matter what precautions are taken, it becomes populated by five billion living bacteria per gram! Some kinds of bacteria, once they are well established in the digestive tract, protect the host against other dangerous bacteria. The resistance which a child has to infectious diseases depends on the presence of some protective bacteria in its digestive tract. Human breast milk has the power to sort out which bacteria will be protective and help them grow. The dominant flora of a breastfed baby is made up of 'lactobacillus bifidus', which is associated with a low level of colibacillus. Even if the 'bifidus factor' is added to humanized milk, the balance of the intestinal flora will still be weighted towards colibacillus, which lowers the acid balance and makes the child more vulnerable to certain pathogenic bacteria.

The intestinal flora can be disturbed from the very start by antibiotics given either to the mother or the baby. All these disturbances are irreversible and can have a permanent effect on the way in which a person will be able to combat bacterial attacks. Discussing the way bacteria settle in the intestines reminds us of the far-reaching importance of the primal period – the time around birth. It is also a cause for regret that most babies are forced to have their first experiences in an environment which is very different from what will be the family environment. Put another way, we are sorry that most babies are born in hospitals where selected germs are particularly dangerous. The time when a baby first meets the world of bacteria corresponds exactly with what is called a sensitive period, a critical period, a short span of time which will never happen again and whose consequences are permanent.

In my view, good health is almost synonymous with a good immune system. In the genesis of good health, one of the essential functions of breastfeeding is to bridge the gap between the time when maternal antibodies are given to the fetus by the placenta, and the time when the child's immune system is completely mature and autonomous. Human breast milk has in it different types of antibodies, but the most important are the secretory antibodies, commonly called IgA. The IgA cover the baby's intestinal wall and protect it against any kind of invasion from pathogenic germs and against any kind of penetration by big molecules to which the baby might become permanently sensitive. These antibodies are different from one mother to another, from one baby to another, and even from one sucking to another. The very individual quality of the antibodies is best seen when the baby has an infection. The baby communicates this infection to the mother while sucking. The breast responds by producing the appropriate antibodies. In this way mother and baby share a kind of mutual protection system. As a living tissue, human breast milk also contains catalysts; enzymes such as the one which aids the digestion of fats after being mixed with bile.

However advanced artificial milk might be, it cannot provide basic nutrients in the same way as human breast milk. As an example, it is only human milk which contains the famous GLA, the direct precursor of prostaglandins 1. When one is aware of the key role of the fatty acids in the maturation of the huge human brain, one can see that this particular quality of human milk merits special attention. One must always remember that the human brain grows from about 450cc up to 1,000cc during the first year of life and that the brain needs very specific fat materials for optimum development. On this point the so-called 'follow on' milks cannot satisfy all the needs of a human baby. They do not contain – or contain little – of the most important fatty acids for building the human brain (areachidonic and docasahexaenoec acid).

## Conclusion

The irreplaceable qualities of human milk indicate that the frequent difficulties in breastfeeding should be considered as a major cause for concern to anyone interested in public health. Difficulties in breastfeeding, just as difficulties in childbirth and sexual difficulties, are diseases of civilization. And each in their turn is creating disease.

Love; sexuality; health. These are words which only our Western analytical brain can consider as separate entities.

# CHAPTER 6

# Social and Religious Instincts

In the same way as emotions are shared, so health is shared. Health is not the attribute of an isolated individual. Every person has a fundamental need; the need to feel that he is integrated into a group, into a community. To live for the group, to survive for the group is part of the need to live, an aspect of the dynamics of survival. The place which an individual has in a group is a factor which influences his health. When you have responsibility your health is better than if you were in a submissive state; in either case your emotional balance, your hormonal balance and your immune system are affected.

## The Need to Live for the Group

There are some apparent contradictions in the various aspects of the dynamics of survival. For example, conflicts and fights between different members of a group might reflect a priority given to individual needs. Sexual competition, the need to survive through procreation, has always imposed limits on the notion of a group. The dynamics of survival for the group can be weakened, leading to selfish behaviour, anti-social behaviour and delinquency. But paradoxically, the dynamics of survival for the group can be stronger than any other needs. The most extreme forms of behaviour – suicide for altruism or patriotism, or kamikaze death – are still subjects for news stories.

In certain spheres of life, human adaptability seems limitless. Human beings have been able to adapt themselves to life in every latitude and every climate; to life by the sea, along river banks and up mountains. There is very little in common between the diets of someone living in Lapland, someone living in New York or someone living in tropical Africa.

On the other hand, human adaptability is very limited when it comes to social needs. By studying a person's social relationships you will have the best indicator of his risks of disease and death. The best predictors of mortality risks are gleaned from statistics which measure things like the number of persons per household and the social activities inside and outside the house. Studies done in Norway, California (Alameda County) and Canada have all shown this. They also demonstrate most eloquently that the first need of every human being is to feel part of a group.

The problem is that the notion of 'group' has undergone considerable evolution in the course of the history of mankind. Human groups of today are more and more difficult to define and, so it seems, have nothing in common with groups in the past. One imagines that in the beginning the human group was not very different from the hunter-gatherer societies which have been studied in depth, such as the Mbuti Pygmies of the tropical rain forest and the Bushmen of the Kalahari Desert. In these societies the men went out to hunt while the women were busy gathering around the camp. Strong ties between males made it possible for them to coexist in the group they were born into until adulthood. It also made it possible for them to hunt and fish in a collective and structured way. To divide and

75

coordinate work in this way is a characteristic of humans. It is likely that in these groups aggression could express itself by hunting big game.

Rivalries and conflicts between human groups have probably always existed. Leaders of war have always used war to reinforce their power. War can be considered as an expression of the dynamics of survival for the group. Human societies have changed considerably over the ages. The introduction of agriculture and the breeding of animals was an important stage. The extended family and the village became basic structures. Then came cities with their districts; counties; provinces; states; nation states; groups of states; superpowers. The notion of what a group is has become more and more blurred, so blurred that the dynamics of survival for the group is apparently disappearing in industrialized man. He is considered an individualist, a narcissist. It is commonplace to claim that antisocial acts and delinquency are on the increase. Delinquency is a kind of disease of our civilization. We are just beginning to see a link between antisocial behaviour and events that happen at the beginning of life, during the primal period.

Despite appearances, this dynamic to survive for the group has not, in fact, been extinguished in our society. For example, during recent wars such as in Algeria, Korea and Vietnam some soldiers belonging to the most industrialized nations were capable of sacrificing their own lives for the group, for example by throwing themselves on to a grenade so comrades could be saved. The dynamic to survive for the group has tended to be underestimated or misunderstood in our society because it always surfaces in a new guise, adapted to completely new conditions.

Traditionally, women belonging to a group helped each other during pregnancy, childbirth and while looking after a baby. It was an essential part of altruistic behaviour. Today, pregnant women still have that strong need to meet

76

other pregnant women and to meet mothers with babies. This explains the rise of various types of groups concerned with preparation for childbirth. Whether women meet each other to swim, or to sing, to do exercises, to talk or to listen, the important thing is that they meet. The places where women give birth might go beyond their original aim and become places where women can help each other during pregnancy and breastfeeding.

Some apparently absurd or irrational behaviour seen nowadays can only be understood as new ways of expressing the dynamic to survive for the group. For example, the popularity of a sport like football is quite astonishing. An important football match has the power to rouse several million television viewers. Looked at rationally, it is amazing that the public, the media and political leaders can give so much importance to the way eleven grown men coordinate their action to make a ball go into a small space called a goal. In fact, a football team is probably very similar to a prehistoric group of humans, who were also capable of structured and coordinated actions in hunting and in war. Apparently human beings are programmed for maximum efficiency when a team has about ten or fifteen people in it.

Humans are programmed to live in small communities. Football match spectators are able to identify themselves with the players on their side. Now and then the game itself is not enough to channel their energies and there are incidents: fights between the players, punch-ups between the supporters, mayhem from supporters on the football pitch. However, football hooliganism is a sociological phenomenon which is very different from delinquency. Delinquency is a sign of a weakened capacity to be part of a group, whereas hooliganism shows a very strong need for social cohesion and group identification which has no other way of expressing itself in daily life. Cohesion of a group

77

depends on loyalty amongst its members and a clear set of objectives of what they want to achieve.

Altruism, like war and indeed like all manifestations of the dynamic to survive for the group, has very deep biological roots. The behaviour of a soldier who sacrifices himself in order to save a group of comrades is not very different from the behaviour of a bee which kills itself by leaving its sting in somebody's skin or of a robin which warns other birds in its flock that a falcon is on its way by using a particular sound, thus risking its own life. Basically, war is not very different from animals fighting for food or territory. The difference is that humans can coordinate, structure and complete their actions.

The difficulty is to know exactly what a human group is these days. There can only be a group where it is possible for the individuals within it to communicate with each other. Communication is not just about exchanging information; it is also about sharing emotions, sharing feelings. The things which cement a group are sympathy, compassion, shared joys, fear. Originally, a group could only be small and was usually rooted in a particular geographical place. But now limitations like that have been shaken up. So people living in different continents can share the same values, the same interests, the same feelings, and together make up real communities without there being any geographical ties. A television viewer in Europe can feel overcome with compassion when he sees an African baby starving to death. With modern communications and an awareness of ecology, humanity as a whole tends to become a group. This being so, wars of the future may be acts of criminality and less groups struggling for their own survival. Perhaps we are reaching a time when war – even economic war – will seem absurd.

# The Religious Instinct

Both altruism and war originate in the most archaic structures of the brain, the primal brain. The same is true of the religious instinct, that vision of the universe which transends time and space and which gives us a sense of belonging to something universal. The religious instinct is universal and cross-cultural. It can be repressed or channelled in different ways both by culture and by churches. No matter what, it always finds ways to express itself. It always reappears, sometimes in surprising ways.

While our upper brain, our neocortex, handles the information given to it by the sense organs and is able to have knowledge of the universe which is limited by time and space, the primal brain goes beyond that, beyond the rational world. Life has been able to develop, evolve and get more complex because the supercomputer contained in the new brain has been at its service. But from the moment this supercomputer becomes overpowerful and represses the primal brain the whole of life will be threatened.

With most people, the religious sense is always there, but hidden. It manifests itself in having beliefs, opinions, in artistic or scientific creativity, in the conviction that powerful creators exist and in a sense of the sacred. Magic, the irrational, the supernatural, the fantastic, fairy tales – people need all these things. People also need to worship. The emotions shared by 70,000 people at a pop concert are also manifestations of the religious sense. It is this religious sense which pushes the philosopher or scientist to search for a unity in universal existence. It is this religious sense which enabled Einstein to elaborate the theory of relativity before demonstrating it mathematically.

Sometimes the religious sense is recognized as such and channelled by the churches. For thousands of years, since the male became aware of his power in fertility the sense of paternity became stronger, and since the rise of the

79

monotheistic religions the religious sense has openly expressed itself by the adoration of an all-powerful father figure.

In some circumstances, the religious sense can reach a climax. Some works of art, some scenery, taking part in some events, some physiological changes in the state of consciousness such as orgasm, childbirth or trance create emotions which bring a sense of eternity, of something infinite, something oceanic. At its most extreme, it is a mystical experience. Mystical experience seems to be as old as mankind itself and the words used to describe it have been numerous: cosmic experience, enlightenment, nirvana, transpersonal experience, transcendental experience, supreme realization, heavenly realm, seventh heaven, mystical ecstacy, peak experience, meeting God, and so on.

This great number of ways to describe mystical experience arises because it involves the emotions and subjective experience which are difficult to communicate in words, and because such experiences have happened in widely diverse cultures. During these mystical experiences a person perceives the unity of the cosmos and himself within it; enlightenment is accompanied by feelings of peace and universal love. A person perceives how insignificant and illusory our world is and he loses the fear of death. A mystical experience is often the result of a long evolution in a person, but can happen at an unexpected time. It marks the beginning of a deep transformation of the individual, who becomes a magnetic attraction to other people.

The religious sense evolves with age. In children it is strong and malleable, and easily directed by the churches. Enlightenments, mystical experiences, often happen between the age of thirty and thirty-five. They seem to correspond to a particular activity of the system of endorphins and perhaps to the ability to disassociate the release of some endorphins from that of other stress hormones. Some spiritual masters have reached the capacity of being

80

able to repeat such experiences. It has been noted that some spiritual masters have big breasts; and we know that endorphins are releasers of prolactin.

The religious sense, the capacity to believe, is not equally developed in every person and in every society. However, obvious good health and long life are both characteristics of particular societies known for their deep religious sense, whether they are Mohammedans as in the case of the Hunzas, Russian Orthodox in the Caucasus or Roman Catholics in Ecuador. Being able to believe makes it easier to fight against disease. Doctors know about the placebo effect. It means that an ill person believes that a medicine will work even if the real medicine has been replaced by a substitute. The religious sense tends to be weaker in a society which neglects the development of the primal brain. Only a sick man, who is losing the feeling that he is part of the universe, could take the process of destroying our earth so far. But if the religious sense comes from the primal brain – the brain which gives us the impetus to survive – as long as there are humans who struggle to live, the religious sense will persist.

'The twenty-first century will be spiritual, or will not be.' (Malraux)

# CHAPTER 7

# The Gardener

Nowadays the fear of stress is like the fear of germs used to be at the beginning of the century. During Pasteur's era, germs became the enemy. Now the word 'hygiene' no longer means a search for health, but just another way of talking about cleanliness. So today stress has replaced germs as the enemy. No one knows exactly what the word stress means; only that it is dangerous. If only we could get rid of the stresses of modern life, there would be a general sense of well being – or so one might think.

But, in fact, we need both bacteria and stress. Some of our organs cannot work properly without bacteria. The door to the world of bacteria opens at birth, and birth is also a spectacular challenge for the stress hormones. Studies have shown that animals who are raised in an environment which is free from any bacteria fall ill and lose all their ability to adapt. It is by confronting bacteria face to face that the immune system transforms itself and acquires its capacity to fight. It is the same story with stress. Any change in the environment which encourages a person's capacity to adapt also transforms him. The effort necessary for this is a creative force. It is the same creative force that works in the fight against bacteria and in the elaboration of new ideas. Highly creative people are often those whose capacities for adaptation have been put to a strong challenge. For example, Hans Selye, before he founded his theories on stress in Montreal, had to leave Prague, change his language and go to another continent!

So the priority is not to eliminate all bacteria, all viruses and all stresses, but to make sure that each person has every chance of being able to develop his capacities for adaptation, in other words to develop his primal adaptive system. The priority is to focus on the period of dependency on the mother.

Later on, primal health can be cultivated. The way each person regards his own health and the way society regards public health may be compared to the way a gardener tends his plants. To be a true gardener one has to be aware of a plant's fundamental requirements and be able to meet them. One also has to be able to adapt to changing circumstances.

## Feeding with Emotions

Feeding the primal adaptive system first of all means feeding it with positive emotions. We know that the system is always in a state of change; whenever there is any change it is an emotion, something which involves the primal brain, the hormonal system and the immune system. Some emotions depress the adaptive systems: situations of helplessness and hopelessness, loss of love, submission, defeat. By contrast, the positive emotions stimulate the adaptive systems: responsibility, control, creativity, victory, new love.

Basic emotional needs can only be met within the context of a group. The place which an individual holds within a group influences his emotional state and his basic mood. Long life or good health into old age often go with having responsibilities or creative activities. No matter what culture a person lives in, daily life cannot always satisfy the need for positive emotions, and does not usually sufficiently challenge a person's creative abilities. People are always searching for ways to overcome these frustrations. One way to do this is through art.

## Art

Art is creation. Art creates emotions. Art makes you want to share emotions; it is a way of communicating. Artistic expression is specifically human and cannot be disassociated from a culture. It implies common conditioning, and common points in the education of the senses. Art has always had close connections with the maintenance of good health and with healing.

The relationship between art and healing is universal. Nowadays we might consider art to be a human endeavour which succeeds in synthesizing the rationality of the new brain and the activity of the primal brain. All art emanates from sensitivity and appeal to sensitivity but, at the same time it demands techniques and means of expression which require training. Each sensory and each physiological function can be the basis of a form of art.

Dancing is one of the most primitive and universal of all art forms. At its roots are functions which give us information about our movements and the position of our body. These basic sensory functions start very early in fetal life, such as the vestibular system situated in the inner ear. The vestibular system plays an important role in balance. Another root of dance is rhythm; and it is well known that these rhythms are often the rhythms of the body, which is why they can be so varied. Perhaps some are like the rhythms of the maternal aorta; others may be reminiscent of the rocking experienced in the womb or later in the mother's arms. Let us take as an example the tempo of Balinese music; it is exactly the same as when the Balinese women pound rice. This may be because Balinese babies spend many hours on their mother's hip while she is pounding the rice.

Movements in dance also have an infinite diversity and can bring about a wide variety of emotional states. These emotional states are transformed and reinforced when people dance together. Some traditional dances lead to states of ecstasy, to collective trance, which means a deep readjustment of the emotional system. In particular, it might be a powerful way of switching on the system of endorphins. Dance is so universal that it can be considered to be a fundamental human need. This need to dance is able to resist all kinds of repression. For example, in France during the German occupation, *Le Bal Defendu* was the title of a famous song inspired by some prohibited dance halls.

The same could be said about singing, which in any case often goes together with dancing. There is no human society where singing is unknown. Darwin thought that singing might have come before articulated language as the human voice has a musical quality when emotions are being expressed. Humans have always heard the sound of lullabies as babies. Through the ages singing has been used to reinforce religious feelings and to help heal the sick. Incantations have always held an important place in rites of magic associated with healing. Some of these incantations are slow, with notes held a long time; others are fast, rhythmic and repetitive. In Indonesia, the traditional medicine men of shamanism sing when they go into the house of a sick person and while they try and find the cause of his illness. In ancient Greece, medical songs were often accompanied by the lyre. Homer told how the Greeks put a stop to the plague by using the power and charm of some special songs called 'epimoimia'. The Greeks thought that fatigue and a lack of zest for life reduced resistance to diseases, while joy and serenity stimulated this resistance. The Greeks were avant-garde about 'psycho-immunology'.

In the Middle Ages, flagellants came on the scene to combat epidemics, the Black Plague in particular. They were made up of groups who travelled round the country singing a special song called *La Lopinette*. During the Renaissance, choral singing developed. It was at this time that Doctor Cornelius Agrippa claimed that singing had a greater power than the sound made by instruments.

Today, there is a tendency to associate the effects of dance, singing and music together. But in fact there is an essential and often overlooked difference between the activity of a dancer and of a singer and the passivity of someone who just listens to music. In our technological society, many people never sing. Instead, they listen to recorded music; they listen to singers through the medium of radio, records, cassettes or television. This is what led Marie Louise Aucher, a former professional singer in France, to create 'psychophonia'. She has spent her whole life helping other people to rediscover singing. She has encouraged adults, children, children with Down's Syndrome and old people. She was the source of singing groups for pregnant women.

These groups are a fruitful way of combining two things: meeting other women and singing. Marie Louise has also been interested in the development of our vibratory sense and the sense of rhythm during life in the womb. Her greatest ambition at the end of her career has been to rehabilitate family singing. She has the extraordinary gift of making emotions shared and, more than that, of inducing a cascade of different emotional states, whether it be serenity, tenderness, pity, surprise, gaity, intense joy or collective ecstasy. She was able to compose the songs in her repertoire thanks to her poetic vision of the universe. There is no dividing line between poetry and singing. Possibly Marie

Louise Aucher has been one of the great therapists of this century.

Since time immemorial, there have always been close ties between health, religion and music. According to the Bible, David entered the court of King Saul to play the sitar and calm the cries of madness of the first king of Israel. For the Greeks, health was order and harmony between body and soul. That is why music, which represents order and harmony, played an important role in the Greek approach to health.

Nowadays the benefits of music therapy are becoming better known, particularly for the treatment of anxiety states, inhibition and behaviour where people give up easily. Music therapy has been used in the treatment of alcoholism; this is done as group therapy, with the help of families and former drinkers. All forms of art, all forms of artistic creativity can be a source of positive emotions. The term 'art therapy' above all makes you think of the visual arts and handicrafts, such as drawing, painting, sculpture, pottery, and so on. An emotion is less pathogenic when it finds a way to express itself. Artistic expression might be a way to compensate for the negative effects of some painful experiences. This is why great suffering and despair have been expressed through art over the ages, and very ill people have found refuge in artistic creativity. The works of Van Gogh cannot be disassociated from his madness. Where would contemporary French literature be without those great asthmatics Gide, Proust, Valery or Mallarmé?

Likewise, the literature of the English language calls forth names such as Lord Byron, who lost his father when he was three years old, was often abused by his mother and had a club foot; Charles Dickens, who had memories of an unhappy childhood; Ernest Hemingway, who witnessed the suicide of his father and was destined to commit suicide himself; Somerset Maugham, who lost his mother when he was eight, his father when he was ten then was sent to

France for health reasons; Virginia Woolf, who first experienced depression when she was thirteen and who committed suicide by drowning; or William Wordsworth, who lost his mother at eight years old and his father at thirteen. A recent British study established a link between intense artistic creativity and manic depression. The most vulnerable were poets. Certainly everybody should do his best to cultivate good health. But good health should not become a moral value; stereotyped good health would deprive society of some of its most creative individuals.


## Therapies

People have always created the means for positive emotions. When the declared objective is to improve health, we call them therapies. The dividing line between art and therapy is vague. Therapy on its own can be considered a form of art. A great therapist, a great healer, is ideally someone in good health who possesses the art of being able to pass on positive emotions by whatever means. The best means are those which are based on fundamental human needs.

Recently, laughter therapy has become the vogue, particularly in the USA, since Norman Cousins told how he had cured himself of a degenerative condition of the spine, partly by watching comic films such as those of the Marx brothers. After an international symposium in Washington, laughter centres were created. So we are just rediscovering what Rabelais knew; as a doctor he was the first to use laughter therapy. Rabelais observed that people who had syphilitic skin eruptions which had been treated with a mercury ointment had little chance of surviving. So he gave these patients his writings to make them laugh – he could not find a more expedient remedy. Even in ancient times, doctors already knew that laughter could strengthen the whole organism, the lungs in particular. In the thirteenth century Henri de Mondeville used laughter to rehabilitate people who had had operations; and Richard Mulcaster, an English doctor living in the sixteenth century, rang the praises of laughter treatment for people with cold hands. Human beings have always laughed, whatever the culture. Collective laughter is something well known by anthropologists whether among the Hopi Indians, the Amazonian Indians or the blacks of the Sudan. Laughter has always been a way to strengthen the group.

True laughter expresses pleasant emotions; it happens when something suddenly takes you by surprise and you stop being serious. Laughing is contagious; laughing is universal. Laughing may not be confined to humans; indeed, apes have been seen to laugh. The brain structures involved in laughter are becoming better known. These seem to be the pleasure centres of the hypothalamus connected with certain precise zones of the right prefrontal cortex. The ability to laugh is destroyed if these zones are damaged. The fact that the laughter centre is situated on the righthand side of the brain means that things which make you laugh have nothing to do with being analytical.

It goes without saying that you don't have to consult a therapist to laugh! There are professional comics, and a great many people who have the ability to make people laugh. When a French opinion poll wanted to know which people could make people laugh the most, one well-known politician came top of the list! The poll also found that only eight per cent of French people laugh more than five minutes a day.

From the beginning of human societies, almost all therapies have been conducted through the intermediary of a therapist, whatever they might have been called – shaman, healer or psychotherapist. Despite the diversity of different cultures, different techniques and, above all, different basic theories, what the various therapies have in common is more striking than their differences. Therapists have always

89

relied on a reduction in control by the neocortex to release emotions. Above everything else, the shamans use their powerful charismatic image in a world where health and medicine are not separated. But they also use techniques which are not so very different from psychodrama, dream analysis, hypnotic suggestion and visualization.

Modern psychotherapists refer to a particular theory when they define their techniques. Conventional psychoanalysts depress the control by the neocortex by techniques such as free association of ideas. Psychoanalytic techniques seem to reactivate those parts of the brain which were particularly active during childhood. As psychoanalysts practise in a society where the nuclear family is the norm, they know a lot about conflicts, such as the Oedipus complex. Other therapists use techniques which depress the control by the neocortex very powerfully, and which stimulate brain zones which were especially active during early stages in the person's life. All therapies inspired by Wilhelm Reich belong to this group, including bio-energetics, vegetotherapy, the primal therapy of Arthur Janov, rebirthing and some modern ways of using hypnosis. These therapies seem to be particularly attractive to people who had a difficult birth, or difficulties around that period . . . people in this category are likely to increase in the future. The emotions released by such therapies are not always pleasant, but then a positive emotion is not always a pleasant one. An emotion which you keep bottled up, for example anger, is more pathogenic inside than when you let it out.

Certain traditional practices have been adapted to the technological and scientific context of the latter part of the twentieth century and share the spirit of the gardener. Transcendental meditation is a good example of this. People are given a mantra – a special and secret word – which they repeat to induce a state of meditation. Another example is biofeedback. With the help of a simple device,

90

the person learns how to control the activity of the brain and to produce an 'alpha' rhythm, the rhythm which corresponds to a feeling of well-being, even bliss. In the same way, some people have adapted visualization techniques which were traditionally used by the yogis to control their visceral functions. Visualization techniques have been used notably against cancer, where the person visualizes his white blood cells attacking the cancer cells. Such techniques have reported better success rates than could have been expected with conventional medicine.

## Environment

The word emotion usually makes you think of changes which do not last long. The maintenance of primal health is also the maintenance of a person's basic mood, which stays the same regardless of events which can trigger strong emotions. Mood is not dependent only on human factors. People also need vegetation and animals to maintain their emotional balance – in other words, their health. Mood also depends on a great many factors which are imperceptible and difficult to analyse, but which are constantly influencing us in our everyday lives.

Colours are probably important elements in our environment. Therapists who use colours say that blue is a relaxing and even creative colour; blue would be the best colour for migraine sufferers or asthmatics. Red is stimulating and exciting; its effects are counterbalanced by green. Orange seems to have anti-depressant qualities and be able to generate feelings of joy. On the other hand, unbroken white seems to be able to bring on feelings of fear and is difficult to put up with for any length of time (and this is the colour usually chosen for hospital walls!).

Of course, the effects of colours depend to a great extent on our individual conditioning. However, it seems that colours are important not just for humans, but for every living thing. This has been demonstrated with plants. Experiments with watercress have shown big differences in the rate of growth, colour, texture, and flavour depending on whether the coloured light they had been under was red, green, white or blue. (The best colour for them was blue.)

Some elements are important too for the emotional system, particularly water. Water has a powerful attraction for all human beings in a variety of different ways. Millions of men spend their leisure time fishing, which means looking at water. Many people spend their holidays on a beach, facing the sea. It seems that the attraction of water is stronger at some times than others, for example during pregnancy and childbirth. Swimming pools which reserve special times for pregnant women become popular very fast. I have never considered birth under water to be an end in itself, but the result of an incredible attraction which water has for some women while they are in labour. Water makes many pregnant women dream; water makes us all dream. Oceans, seas, waves, springs, rivers, streams, fountains – all these are essential themes in poetry. Experts in the valuation of paintings first want to know if there is any water in the picture – it raises the value!

Water has always been used for healing. There is a wide range of therapies which use water. Even though there is no solid basis to their theories, water therapies nevertheless continue to multiply and to help many people, with many types of hydrotherapy, balneotherapy, spas, thalassotherapy, flotation tanks, and so on.

In every civilization, water has always been the symbol of mother, and sick people have always needed a feminine and maternal environment. In ancient Greece, health was symbolized by a female goddess, Hygieia, and the secrets of healing were first of all guarded by priestesses. It was not until a patriarchal social order was well established that

Hygieia became the daughter of a God, Aesculape, father of all doctors. The art of healing in the bosom of the family has always been a female prerogative, a motherly task. Even in our big modern hospitals, which are dominated by male doctors, female nurses continue to play an essential role.

There is, of course, a great deal more to be said about how the environment can affect health. Everybody searches for beauty in their lives, whether in architecture, scenery or in material objects inside their homes. 'A thing of beauty is a joy forever.'

## Exercise

It is certainly not by chance that some activities which can satisfy several basic human needs at the same time have developed so quickly during the twentieth century. Sport satisfies both the need for play and for physical exercise. Games have always been a way to feed human beings with positive emotions. It is said the Romans wanted nothing more than bread and games.

It is commonplace to emphasize the benefits of exercise and the ill effects of a sedentary life. The need for exercise varies according to the training acquired during childhood and adolescence, and to age and sex. It is obvious that most people nowadays are not active enough in their daily lives. Others dangerously overestimate their possibilities. The health risks connected with sport are becoming better known. The warning signals appear when the sportsman goes beyond certain limits. One example is women who stop menstruating during intensive training. Sport is much more than simply a way of satisfying the need for physical exercise; it is also a way to experience those emotions which go with victory or defeat. With the same amount of energy spent, the emotional gains from winning a football match

93

cannot be compared with losing against the clock after running ten times round an empty stadium.

Our muscular activity, our emotional state and our mood determine at any given moment our supply of oxygen – in other words they affect how we breathe. The rhythm and depth of our breathing depend on emotions and exercise. But, naturally, the air we breathe differs according to the climate and the extent of industrialization.

## Food

Cultivating the primal adaptive system means not only supplying positive emotions and oxygen; it also means feeding it in the literal sense of the word. The importance of nutrition has been the subject of countless articles, books, television and radio programmes – so much so that good health is sometimes synonymous with healthy nutrition. What we eat in our daily life has become an obsession for some people. One can easily forget that the good or bad effects of a meal depend on factors other than just the composition of the food. Eating is also a way of stimulating the basic senses of taste and smell. The sense of smell is a very special sensory function because it connects directly with the part of the primal brain called the 'limbic system'. Even though the sense of smell is less developed in man than it is in some other mammals, its role is probably underestimated. For example, an underdeveloped olfactory tract goes together with a very low level of circulating sex hormones. A meal is also a social event, something to share, a way of communicating with other people, a communion.

The most important nutritional thing is water. The priority for public health is the supply of water that is safe to drink. The French king Dagobert deserves to be remembered better than just for a funny song. He introduced an order in the year AD 630 which condemned anyone who fouled the public fountains. Perhaps he did more for his subjects than all the doctors in his kingdom. What we have to fear nowadays in the industrialized countries is chemical pollution, rather than pollution by bacteria. Once the need for drinkable water is met, humans are able to adapt to many different kinds of food after the period in their lives when all they need is breast milk.

A lack of food depresses our systems of adaptation. The connection between famines and epidemics has been known for centuries. Some diseases are the equivalent of food deficiencies and go together with a lowering of the body's defences; for example, some types of nephrosis, which involve a massive loss of proteins in the urine, or some cancers or alcoholism. Even today, famines still occur in tropical countries, such as Ethiopia. When children get kwashiorkor, a serious form of malnutrition, the death rate from infectious diseases such as measles or gastro-enteritis rises. This malnutrition causes the thymus and lymphoid tissues to atrophy and also depresses the role of the T lymphocytes. The level of antibodies in the blood does not go down; on the contrary it stays high because of the many infections. But the synthesis of local antibodies (IgA) which protect the walls of the intestines and the respiratory tract is lowered. The polynuclear white cells – that is those which have the capacity to encircle and destroy micro-organisms – stop being aggressive. Malnutrition brings with it lesions in the skin and the mucous membranes, which are the first protective barriers.

In the industrialized countries the standard of living is high enough for most individuals' need for food to be met. The improvement in nutrition, both in quantity and variety, is one of the factors which helps explain the increase in height and lifespan. But despite everything, twentieth century man has not fully exploited the potential for nutrition at his disposal. Moreover, extreme poverty exists even within the richest nations.

There are certainly many harmful habits where food is concerned; bad habits which are being practised on a huge scale. Some of these habits originated with techniques that are so old that we would not dare question them. The first of these is cooking. The bad effects of cooking have gone unsuspected for a long time, but there are in fact many of them. The most dangerous is probably heating certain oils at a high temperature. Our body needs essential fatty acids which come from leaves and seeds, from the meat of animals which eat plants, and from fish. In the language of biochemistry essential fatty acids are biologically active when the molecules are in what is known as the 'cis' form. When heated at a high temperature, the molecules in these fatty acids change their shape from the 'cis' form to the 'trans' form, which blocks the metabolism of essential fatty acids vital to the body. Essential fatty acids not only go into the making of cell membranes and play a role in the synthesis of cholesterol, but they are also necessary for the synthesis of prostaglandins. Moreover, at a high temperature the molecules of the unsaturated fatty acid more easily accept atoms of oxygen. This process is called oxidation. These atoms of oxygen can later detach themselves and latch onto another molecule. These dangerous unstable oxygen-carrying molecules are called free radicals. They can set up destructive chain reactions which damage cells and probably play a role in the origin of diseases like cancer and arteriosclerosis.

Cooking also transforms proteins. Some amino acids such as lysine and cystine are particularly vulnerable. Cooking destroys many enzymes, the living catalysts, and therefore changes the way food is digested. Some vitamins are particularly fragile (vitamins B and C). Cooking also has the effect of conditioning the sense of taste very easily, and contributes to an altered food instinct.

The second big group of innovative techniques is the development of agriculture and breeding which took place at the time of the Neolithic revolution – about ten thousand years ago. It has been shown that the average height of man decreased by fifteen centimetres after the beginning of agriculture both in Europe and on the continents of America. There are many reasons for this. The development of agriculture modified family structures and the relationship between men and women in general, in such a way that the life of pregnant women and young mothers was transformed; and thus the life of babies in the primal period. At the same time, eating habits radically changed. The plants people ate became less varied. Their diet contained more starch and less proteins with the cultivation of vegetables. The amount of fibrous vegetables decreased. Animals reared on a farm became bigger than their ancestors and the composition of their fat became transformed.

The meat of wild animals contains an appreciable quantity of a polyunsaturated, long-chain fatty acid (eicosapentanoeic acid) which protects against arterial damage. No trace of this fatty acid can be found in beef. The meat of farm animals has more calories for less protein. Agriculture and breeding have also considerably modified the balance between minerals and vitamins.

It was not until the industrial revolution that the next spectacular change in our eating habits took place with the development of the food industry. It became easier and easier to get pure sugar. Sugar is a big factor in dental caries; it penetrates very quickly into the bloodstream after having been absorbed by the intestines, and tends to overwork the pancreas which secretes insulin. It disturbs the synthesis of GLA, precursor of prostaglandins 1.

The processing of oils and margarines since the 1920s introduced into the market a large amount of trans fatty acids, that is those which block the metabolism of essential fatty acids. Treated milk brought with it a considerable increase in the consumption of dairy products, which means products with saturated fats. Perhaps this might be

97

compensated for by the advances in the transportation and distribution of fish, which is a good source of certain essential fatty acids.

The twentieth century development of the fertilizer industry has also made intensive farming easier. But the exhaustion of soils has robbed much vegetation of certain important minerals, the best example of which is zinc. The nutrition of modern man is deficient in zinc. It is worth mentioning that wheat without its husk contains only 17 per cent of the zinc content of whole wheat. We know that zinc is an essential catalyst in certain metabolic chains, in particular that of essential fatty acids and the synthesis of prostaglandins. The need for zinc is increased by the consumption of sugar, alcohol and the contraceptive pill; it is essential for wound and bone healing. In addition to these inventions and innovations should be added the modern methods of feeding cattle with cereals rather than grass, as this raises even higher the level of saturated fat in the meat found in our butchers' shops today.

It seems that when you put together the introduction of cooking, agriculture and breeding, the rise in the food industries and the changes in the meat we eat, the nutrition of technological man is seriously affected. It is altered in such a way that it magnifies the most common dysfunctions of the primal adaptive system. Obviously, it would be simplistic to suggest that all the different aspects of *the* disease of civilization are a consequence of imbalanced nutrition alone. That would be to ignore the primal period and to overestimate the possibilities of a purely nutritional approach towards disease.

'Homo omnivorous' has a great ability to adapt his eating habits and no one can evaluate precisely all the consequences of dietary habits which science considers harmful. Most people can probably cope with an imperfect diet thanks to a good *terrain*. My mother sums up this point by saying: 'Butter cannot be so bad; I have been eating it every day for ninety years.'

However, many people in our society, especially those who are suffering from any form of *the* disease of civilization, should reduce their intake of animal fat and eat more raw vegetables, more fish and even take some mineral and vitamin supplements, such as zinc. Also, we now know how to take GLA directly (evening primrose oil, blackcurrants, a primitive alga called spirulina). Such an approach fits in well with the attitude of the gardener, who first of all tries to satisfy fundamental needs to the best of his abilities.

When we think of the fundamental needs of technological man, we always have to keep in mind the hunter-gatherer who lived twenty to thirty thousand years ago and who was no different from us genetically. We must always refer to him when we question our limits of adaptability and also our potential. Whether we are talking about the development of the primal adaptive capacities, or about the maintenance of a basic state of health, there is no doubt that humans do have a potential which is as yet both unsuspected and unexploited.

# CHAPTER 8

# The Doctor

The history of medicine often seems like the history of new treatments. They arrive on the scene, are widely accepted and used, and are then condemned and disappear because the side-effects outweigh their advantages. This was already true in the time of Molière. During his epoch, however, the arsenal of treatments was limited. There was, for example, blood-letting, and drugs like antimony. Nobody will ever be able to estimate the harm done by blood-letting and antimony. Because Louis XIV thought he had been cured by antimony, it was not until two centuries later that it became completely discredited in France!

The history of medicine can only be understood properly when you compare the typical attitudes of a doctor with those of a gardener. On the one hand, the gardener cultivates his plants, looks after their health and makes sure that all their needs are met. On the other hand, the doctor who maybe a much more educated man, thinks he can substitute physiological functions with drugs, surgery or irradiation. Of course, this comparison between the gardener and the doctor is simplified as well as being provocative; there are indeed aggressive gardeners, just as there are caring doctors whose first concern is to nurture their patients.


## Drugs

During the twentieth century things have been moving very fast. In the last few decades the rich nations have spent an enormous amount of energy and money on researching new drugs, evaluating their short-term effects, making them, marketing them, using them and then forgetting them. In due course most of the drugs which were designed to fight various aspects of *the* disease of civilization have been found not to withstand the test of time. What also typifies *the* disease of civilization is the inability of modern pharmacology to cure it.

There have been some spectacular drug withdrawals from the market. Everyone knows about Thalidomide, the drug which was aimed at relieving morning sickness in pregnant women. It took several years to discover the link between horrifying abnormalities in babies' limbs and the taking of this drug during pregnancy. Many people remember the story of DES, a synthetic oestrogen which was supposed to prevent miscarriage. Many women took it during the 1940s and early 1950s. It took several years before a clever team in Boston discovered that girls born to mothers who had taken DES in pregnancy often had abnormalities in the cervix and vagina, and had a higher risk of getting cancer of the vagina. The mothers who took DES probably had a greater risk of getting breast cancer. On top of all this, the drug was absolutely useless in preventing miscarriage.

The history of Phisohex (hexaclorophene) is another example of a sensational withdrawal. It is well known that the concentration of ill patients in hospitals together with the widespread use of antibiotics is the perfect breeding ground for bacteria such as staphyloccocus, which can become particularly vigorous and dangerous. Phisohex was a local treatment whose aim was to kill the most common bacteria. When many premature babies died of 'vacuolar encephalopathy', a degeneration of the brain, it was discovered that Phisohex was absorbed by the skin and was toxic to the nervous system. A whole generation of surgical teams had washed their hands in Phisohex for many years. In France there was a famous trial involving a well known brand of talcum powder. This followed the death of four children and the paralysis of two others as a result of using this talc, which contained hexaclorophene.

Much more worrying than the appearance and spectacular disappearance of some drugs is the withdrawal of drugs which have been used for a long time on a huge scale by countless numbers of people suffering from common diseases. A review of the withdrawal of such drugs is also a look back over all the common diseases and the drugs prescribed for them. Many of these drugs had a very wide distribution, often amounting to several million prescriptions a year.

The main reason for these failures is that doctors always want to suppress symptoms without considering that they are the body's way of defending itself. A symptom is a sign of the effort which the body is making to heal itself. So it is harmful to try and reduce a fever; fever is a form of defence. When you have the 'flu the most irrational thing to do is to try and reduce the temperature. Fever does more than protect you against viruses. I once met a Japanese woman by the name of Tokiko Yoshimoto. She described to me how she had had a miraculous escape in a district of Hiroshima where there were no survivors after the atomic bomb was dropped in 1945. At the time of the explosion she was in bed with a strong fever; her defence mechanisms were already in action.

The treatment of hypertension is a good example of how modern pharmacology has failed in the diseases of civilization. A hypertensive person is someone who needs to secrete more adrenalin than normal to face the problems of daily life and to enjoy life's pleasures. It is his way of finding some balance. But what does the doctor do? He either reduces the level of adrenalin with drugs like Aldomet, or he blocks the nerves which increase the activity of the heart pump with drugs called beta-blockers, or he reduces the fluid in the body with diuretics. Nowadays the adverse side-effects of hypertensive drugs are better known. They may be one of the main causes of drug-induced illness in old people. The use of these drugs can only be justified in some serious cases.

A large-scale European study looked at the consequences of long-term treatment of hypertension among patients over sixty years of age. They found a significant lowering of mortality from cardiovascular accidents compared with a group who had had no treatment. But the important point to note is that the overall mortality rate was not lowered. Such a study could not compare the quality of life in the two groups; in general, all the major studies which examine treatments for hypertension are only concerned with the risks of heart attack or stroke.

The common side-effects of Aldomet are depression, fatigue, feeling sleepy and oedema. Its efficiency decreases after some months of treatment so that the dose has to be stepped up. Other side-effects are also coming to light, such as sexual impotence, jaundice and a higher risk from general or local anaesthetic, even including dental treatment.

Beta-blockers, which have been prescribed for millions of people with hypertension all over the world, carry their own risks. The main one is what happens if the patient suddenly stops taking the drug; he could suffer a fatal cardiac arrest. Some of the beta-blockers have been withdrawn because they might be carcinogenic. Diuretics also

103

have undesirable side-effects by disturbing the metabolism of potassium and of fats.

While pharmacologists and doctors search for the ideal hypertensive drug, people outside the field of clinical medicine have approached the problem by turning the traditional thinking upside down. Studies which looked at workers with hypertension suggested that the healthiest were those who did not know they had hypertension and who were not receiving any treatment. Depression is a general characteristic of hypertensives receiving treatment. Sometimes just by giving the diagnosis you can do as much harm as by giving the treatment.

Rabelais, without any device to measure blood pressure but with his laughing therapy, perhaps did more to help hypertensives than the most learned of modern experts. Hypertensives often have other anomalies too, such as raised cholesterol. The simplistic approach is to prescribe a drug which lowers cholesterol. This is why millions of people in the Western world have taken Clofibrate, a drug which effectively lowers cholesterol. But the disadvantage of this drug is that it does not prevent heart disease; and it does increase the risk of gall stones. Today it is advised that this drug should only be used in exceptional circumstances.

The different forms of rheumatism are another example of the failure of modern pharmacology. In the 1950s gold injections were used before people were aware of their toxicity. Then along came cortisone, a miracle medicine, which was going to relieve millions of sufferers. But it only took a few years before a large catalogue of side-effects became apparent: bone fractures due to lack of calcium, necrosis of the head of the femur, moon face, uncontrollable body hair growth, mental disturbances, cataracts and, above all, a depression of the immune system thereby weakening resistance to infections and very likely to cancers.

People thought that it would be possible to replace cortisone with synthetic drugs which had the same properties (corticosteroids). But little by little it became clear that their undesirable side-effects far outweighed any possible benefits, except in very specific acute forms of rheumatism. The fashion of injecting corticosteroids directly into joints lasted barely more than a decade.

At the same time as the corticosteroids, the non-steroidal anti-inflammatory drugs (NSAIs) also appeared on the scene. These drugs suppress inflammatory symptoms, but they do not belong to the same chemical family as corticosteroids. The adverse side-effects of these drugs were rapidly discovered, in particular an increase in arterial pressure, swelling of the ankles, stomach ulcers and blood disorders such as aplastic anaemia.

But it is only since it was found out exactly how they work that their true dangers have become apparent. NSAIs inhibit the synthesis of prostaglandins 1 and 2. This means that the full range and extent of their long-term side effects are difficult to estimate. After having been used for more than two decades on tens of millions of people all over the Western world, these drugs have been almost completely condemned.

There remains aspirin*. The dangers of aspirin for people with chronic illnesses went unsuspected for a long time. Taking aspirin can make the digestive tract bleed and bring on an ulcer. High doses of aspirin are dangerous for the ear. Aspirin interferes with blood clotting. People with allergies or gout should not take aspirin. Pregnant women increase the risk of haemorrhage in the baby. In France there is a saying which goes, 'If you have rheumatism, you'll have a long life.' Maybe this is no longer true thanks to modern medicine.

Fortunately, some people with rheumatism have escaped the conventional attitude and have instead put their faith

* Aspirin appears to inhibit the production of prostaglandins of the series 2 called Thromboxane A2.

in gardener-doctors who still know how to use treatments like thermal cures, baths, heat treatments, different forms of physiotherapy, diets and the healing qualities of the doctor himself.

The abdomen is said to be the sounding board of the emotions. It is not surprising that modern man, whose emotional system is maladjusted from the primal period, should consume so many drugs for the digestive system. For many years gastroenterologists and general practitioners wrote out millions of prescriptions for bismuth salts to reduce acidity in the stomach. Then suddenly, around 1982, countries like France, Switzerland and Australia said that the toxicity was too high compared with the benefits and they recommended that the drug should be withdrawn from use. As early as 1860, Antoine Béchamp warned medical practitioners about the toxicity of bismuth salts and suggested that they should come under the toxic drug regulations.

Drugs which have aluminium hydroxide as their base have also been used on a huge scale for stomach complaints. Their repeated use interferes with the absorption of vitamins and causes a loss of calcium from the bones by forming insoluble phosphates in the digestive tract. Fortunately these insoluble phosphates cannot get into the bloodstream easily, so the risk of aluminium toxification is low. In fact, all these drugs, like all antacids, have a short-term action, followed by a rebound effect with a sudden relapse. It is now admitted that these drugs should not be used, especially not for stomach and duodenal ulcers.

There has been a succession of drugs for stomach ulcers over the last thirty years, one regularly following another as the drug in vogue. It is impossible to mention all of them, from intravenous injections of proteins, to liquorice, to Tagamet. The fashions have not been identical in every country – Tagamet is the most recent anti-ulcer drug to have been used all over the world. This drug does reduce the symptoms of an ulcer but it does not cure it any better than any other drug which a doctor tells you will work. Gastroenterology is one of the areas where the way in which a drug is prescribed is more important than the drug itself. Most patients treated with Tagamet relapse after stopping treatment. Already long-term side-effects are beginning to show up, such as a lowering of male sex hormones in men. The next drug in vogue might be Misoprostol, which is an equivalent of prostaglandins 1. Its aim is to reinforce the defence mechanisms of the mucous membrane in the stomach.

Tranquillizers and anti-depressive drugs have a huge market at the moment. There are two different approaches among practitioners, one in opposition to the other as far as behavioural problems are concerned. On the one hand, there are those practitioners with a leaning towards psychotherapy who tend to exclude the use of drugs and at the same time are not interested in the chemistry of the brain. On the other hand, some practitioners who consider themselves scientific devote all their energy to keeping up with the latest developments in neurophysiology and the science of neurotransmitters. They hope to correct brain chemistry by drugs alone.

What is rare is to find practitioners who are at the same time fully aware of modern neurophysiology and biochemistry, but are also convinced that the use of drugs to modify behaviour is perhaps what a sorcerer's apprentice would do to solve short-term problems without taking into account the infinite complexity of the neuro-hormonal processes. This last group of practitioners know that behavioural problems, some types of anxiety and some kinds of madness are in fact defence reactions which must be respected rather than masked. They also know that emotions are a way to modify brain chemistry and that emotional states are influenced more than anything by the social environment.

Valium is the star among drugs which modify behaviour.

Valium is the most widely prescribed drug in the world. The number of prescriptions amounts to tens of millions. More women take it than men. Valium is the best known in one huge family of tranquillizers (the benzodiazepines). The balance sheet for Valium might have been good if it had only been used in very special cases. But the massive use of the drug has had negative consequences which are impossible to calculate.

When it was first introduced at the beginning of the 1960s Valium was heralded as being a drug which did not create any dependency, whose action did not lessen as time went on and which could be discontinued abruptly without any harmful effects. Now the major worry about Valium is that it does create dependency, its effectiveness does go down within a few weeks, and there are serious withdrawal symptoms if it is stopped suddenly. We not only know that Valium creates dependency, but we are beginning to understand the mechanisms for this.

There are probably receptors in the brain which are sensitive to Valium, just as there are receptors for chemical messengers like morphine. And just as the drug morphine can take the place of endorphins (the body's own morphine) at the corresponding receptors, so Valium can take the place of the body's own physiological tranquillizers.

It is impossible to go into all the ups and downs of all the tranquillizers and anti-depressive drugs. Instead, we will settle for one simple anecdote. In 1983 a pharmaceutical company introduced into the French market an antidepressant drug called Indalpine. The qualities of this new drug were acclaimed, so much so that the Galien Prize was awarded to it in that year and it was prescribed to nearly a million French people. In July 1984 the company who made the drug sent a letter to every doctor asking them to prescribe this drug only to young people who were suffering severe depression. In July 1985 the manufacture of Indalpine was stopped because of its toxicity.

This list of drugs which have been discovered, acclaimed, widely used and later discredited or dropped is an arbitrary one. I could have talked about the use of diuretics during pregnancy; or about all the creams and ointments containing corticosteroids for skin complaints; or I could have talked about the dangers of drugs for asthma. The story of antibiotics and how they have lost their power from overuse is so well known there is no point in saying any more about it. Resistance to the best known synthetic penicillin (Ampicillin) has increased by 28 per cent in thirty years. And in the interests of keeping things simple, I prefer not to discuss drug interactions. It has become too complicated for the human brain!

Most of the drugs which have withstood the test of time were discovered more than thirty years ago. Despite appearances to the contrary, the relationship between medicine and pharmacology has been comparatively barren in recent years. Insulin, which transformed the lives of diabetics, was discovered in 1922; sulphonamides to cure infections were introduced in 1935; Heparin, the first anti-coagulant, came along in 1937; penicillin was introduced in 1941; anti-malarial drugs of the chloroquine family in 1943; streptomycine in 1944; chloramphenicol, mostly used for typhoid, in 1947; vitamin B12 for pernicious anaemia in 1948; the first tetracyclin in 1948; isomazide, the most powerful drug against tuberculosis in 1951; and the first modern tranquillizer in 1952.

Most doctors, and the majority of the general public, are not prepared to make the necessary *prise de conscience* to look at the story of drugs in the way I have described in this chapter. They are constantly being shown the droplets of success, for example the successful use of new drugs for certain blood diseases such as leukemia, or drugs which make organ transplants possible. They tend to forget the ocean of ravages caused by the massive consumption of drugs which can do nothing to restore health to the sick in our civilization. The problem is all the more difficult because the side-effects of drugs usually appear much later and show up in unexpected ways which are difficult to recognize and beyond the comprehension of doctors who are not prepared to understand that health and social structures form a whole.

One such example is fertility drugs, which have made possible the birth of triplets, quadruplets, quintuplets and even sextuplets. Many people have heard about the Lawson quintuplets who were born in New Zealand in 1965. This was the first multiple pregnancy after the introduction of fertility pills. However, not many people are aware of the tragic outcome of this story. The parents divorced and the mother later committed suicide, together with her second husband. There is another similar case that few people know about. William Kienast, the father of quintuplets born in New Jersey, committed suicide shortly after their birth. In northern California alone there were three murders in 1984 in families with multiple births, including the murder of a baby. A London pediatrician, who wrote a book about twins, remarked on the absence of studies about children of multiple pregnancies; no one was asking to what extent such children were affected by brain and motor handicaps.

Only a rapid awareness of the dangers can avoid a repetition of similar mistakes in the near future. It is also possible to make people more aware of some of the dead-ends of modern medicine. For example, today we have drugs like Cyclosporin which can depress the immune system, particularly the function of the T lymphocytes. When this drug is used appropriately it stops transplanted organs from being rejected. So for the time being the balance sheet of Cyclosporin can be considered in its favour. When your only hope is an organ transplant, then you are prepared to put up with Cyclosporin's side-effects such as hypertension, altered sensations, superfluous hair,

110

tremors, swelling of the gums and increased risks of the lymph nodes swelling.

But the danger is that this type of drug has already spread to other areas. It is already beginning to be used in that huge field – auto-immune diseases. When someone has an auto-immune disease it means that the immune system is hitting the wrong target; instead of attacking foreign substances, it attacks some of the body's own cells instead. The reasoning behind using drugs like Cyclosporin is simple (or simplistic): if we depress the immune system then the immune system will not be able to attack the body any longer. When you consider the tendency to announce the triumphs publicly, the dangers are great. Without long-term studies, Cyclosporin has been used for rheumatoid arthritis, for diabetes, for ulcerative colitis, for psoriasis, for lupus, for multiple sclerosis and for AIDS. The market potential for this is quite fantastic.

However, not everyone suffering from an auto-immune disease is happy to go along with this kind of attitude. Some have preferred to adopt the attitude of the gardener. Some people, for example with multiple sclerosis, try and cultivate their own health. They reduce their intake of animal fat; they take supplements of GLA in the form of evening primrose oil; they take various mineral and vitamin supplements such as zinc and the B vitamins. When they tell a member of the medical establishment that they have been well for, say, ten years they are told it proves nothing: a chronic disease such as MS is known for its relapses and sometimes long remissions, and in any case double blind placebo controlled trials would be the only scientific way to prove whether certain treatment worked. Such attitudes put into sharp focus the differences between the gardener and the doctor.

# Surgery

The way in which our society uses surgery also reflects the common mental images associated with the words health and disease. The simplistic view of surgery is that in order to recover health, all you have to do is cut out the disease. I myself have spent much of my life taking out appendices, gall bladders, stomachs, colons, wombs, ovaries, breasts, haemorrhoids, varicose veins, thyroids. It was during the short part of my surgical career spent in the third world, and when I began as a surgeon in a small French town that I felt most satisfaction that I was doing something useful. An overworked surgeon is certainly useful; not only because he is well trained, but also because he only has time to do essential surgery, such as acute appendicitis, burst spleens, ectopic pregnancies, perforated ulcers, strangulated hernias or hernias which are susceptible to strangulation, stones in the bile duct and broken bones.

Things deteriorate when the number of surgeons begins to multiply. There are several reasons why the amount of surgery done has been increased to a worrying degree. Surgeons have to maintain their own skills and the skills of their teams; they have to justify their own existence; they have to earn a good living; they have to satisfy their need to operate. Many studies have shown that for a given population, the number of surgical interventions depends more than anything else on the number of surgeons and the equipment available to them. The costs of surgery are always underestimated. People do consider the risk of death from an operation and the complications which can arise afterwards. But what they never think of is that every surgical intervention puts the adaptive system to the test, whether it is the adrenal glands or the whole immune system. It is difficult to establish a link a long time after an operation between a viral illness or a cancer and surgery which challenged the immune system. Even though some

112

connections have been found, such as a greater risk of cancer of the colon after a gall bladder operation, generally speaking, no connections are ever made.

It would probably be possible in many Western countries to reduce the number of operations without in any way compromising the public's health. It would also be possible to make surgery less complicated. In 1969 I did a review of cases of perforated duodenal ulcers which I had treated by simply 'plugging the hole'. At that time the usual approach was to take advantage of the chance to do a radical intervention, which meant taking out the stomach or cutting the vagal nerves. I found that only one patient in twenty-three needed a second operation. My conclusion was that the nature of the emergency intervention was less important than the way the patient had been nursed – or mothered – during his stay in hospital at a time when he was suffering great anguish.

The rise in the number of surgeons has brought with it not just an increase in the number of operations, but also a never-ending array of new interventions. Some of them, such as total hip replacement, do a lot of good in particular cases when the handicap is weighed up against the risks of infection. But for the most part, however, the story of new surgical procedures can be compared with the story of new drugs.

The saga of coronary artery surgery is a good example of this. At the end of the 1950s, the fashion was to section the internal mammary arteries. This technique lasted up to the time when a couple of surgeons did a study on it. In one group they opened the chest wall without cutting the arteries; in the other group they cut the arteries. They found that the results were exactly the same in the two groups. A little later on, the coronary by-pass operation became common. A vein is taken from the leg and used as a graft to by-pass the obstruction in the coronary artery. This is now a very common operation, and the overall cost

113

of each such operation is estimated at around £15,000. It is estimated that $2.1 billion were spent in the USA in 1984 just for coronary by-pass operations. However, no study has ever proved that this operation increases life expectancy. In May 1985 the Metropolitan Life Insurance Company stated that only 11 per cent of its employees who were under fifty-five were still working five years later after having had coronary by-pass operations.

The time has come to develop other techniques. Angioplasty is now in the process of being used on a large scale. A thin catheter with a balloon is introduced up to the arterial obstruction. The balloon is inflated for a few seconds to open the artery walls. Such a technique makes it possible for a patient to return home and go back to work very quickly. We know that in about 25 per cent of cases, the operation must be repeated within a year, and also that it cannot be used in cases where there are multiple obstructions. An estimated 185,000 angioplasty operations will be performed in 1989. The materials used in each angioplasty cost about $1,000. This income allows the firm which manufactures the catheters to prepare for the next stage, which might be laser surgery.

We might tell the same kind of story about the surgical operation which has been regularly performed to prevent the relapse of a stroke. It is a serious problem when you consider that the stroke is the third largest cause of death and disability in the West. Thousands of people throughout the world had an 'extracranial-intracranial arterial by-pass' between 1969 and 1985. This operation calls for considerable expertise and training in microvascular techniques. Then, an international study, which cost $9,000,000, compared the outcome of 700 patients who underwent surgery after a stroke and 700 patients who did not. The result was that such an operation does not protect against a relapse . . .

The use of radiation might have been another way to

114

illustrate the typical medical approach compared with the gardener approach, as radiation is sometimes used for benign conditions such as acne or warts. But the story would be no different from that of drugs or surgery, so no more needs to be said about it.

## Diagnostic Investigations

My analysis comparing the doctor with the gardener might also include mania for diagnostic tests. The risks involved in some diagnostic tests are rarely balanced against the expected benefits. For example, it has been said that five to ten per cent of cancers in European and American children are connected with the X-rays which pregnant women were given during the 1950s and 1960s.

The risks to life inherent in the exploration of arteries (of the brain, heart, internal organs and limbs) depend to a great extent on how experienced the teams are. In fact, the risks are often underestimated. It is the same for any kind of endoscopy, procedures which make it possible to look inside the human body by introducing a tube either through an orifice or the skin. There are as many kinds of endoscopies as there are natural orifices, hollow organs or natural cavities. Some endoscopies are used in daily practice, such as gynaecological laparoscopy, which consists of introducing a tube across the abdominal wall to see the womb, the fallopian tubes and the ovaries. To be able to see well you have to inflate the abdominal cavity with a gas and put the woman facing head down, commonly with a general anaesthesia. The risk to life of this procedure is disproportionate. Such an investigation should be used only in very exceptional circumstances and then only performed by teams who have the ability to follow up with the most complex abdominal procedures, immediately if necessary.

The madness of investigations can reach such

115

proportions that it defies belief. For example, before dying at the age of forty-two days in a prestigious neonatology unit, one baby underwent 100 X-rays and 300 blood tests.

## Technology out of Control

Paradoxically, it is in intensive care units that one finds the spirit of the gardener-doctor. When the patient is in a critical, or even a catastrophic condition, the doctor's approach is often a long way from the typical medical one. In circumstances like these, the priority is not to make a precise diagnosis or give a specific treatment, but to meet the basic needs while waiting for the patient's autonomy to return.

But it is a different matter when the intensive care unit is specialized. Take, for example, a coronary care unit. In cases where there are no problems with the heart rhythm, there can be no justification for a patient who has suffered a heart attack to be taken systematically to an intensive care unit. No one can say whether by staying at home with the family, with a twice daily injection of Heparin, and without the stress of a ride in the ambulance or of adapting to an unfamiliar place, a patient's chances would be increased or decreased. There are no studies to prove anything either way.

Specialized intensive care units is one example among many of technology out of control. During the 1970s, when I was writing *Entering The World*, my essential theme was the loss of control of technology by the medical institution in the field of childbirth. It took only one decade before this view was shared by some commentators who are part of the medical establishment. A first stage was to consider modern medicine as a luxury hard to afford. 'Medical care is a luxury' was the first phrase of an editorial in *The Lancet*. And now Madame Escoffier-Lambiotte, medical editor of

*Le Monde*, is waiting for the time when we can 'give a compass to the drunken boat of medical technology'. Let us hope that this compass does not take on the shape of an institution which would demand huge sums of money to evaluate techniques which are already obsolete.

What we are waiting for is a radical change of attitude. What happens now when someone falls ill is that a doctor immediately begins treating him with substitutes for his own body's defence system; such as antibiotics, hormones, synthetic drugs, surgery or radiation. These treatments should only be used as an absolutely last resort. We need to multiply the number of 'gardeners' and reduce the number of 'doctors'.

# CHAPTER 9

# Research in Primal Health

The mental pictures commonly associated with the word health guide research programmes. But the new concept of primal health, which turns these mental pictures upside down, might open up a huge field of investigation and might even change priorities. At the moment we are prisoners of outdated mental images and this explains why research is so limited and relatively sterile.

I do not want to say that there has never been any study which brought the importance of the primal period to light. On the contrary, I would like to give some examples of studies which deserve to be included under 'research in primal health'. But they are few and far between, and most of them have escaped notice or have been poorly exploited. In addition to this, the conventional mental pictures are powerfully reprinted every day and everywhere.

If you open any newspaper or look at advertisements on the hoardings, you will be convinced that if only more money were donated, every disease could be eliminated one by one as soon as their cause and cure were discovered. For example, one advertisement which appears frequently in British newspapers and on hoardings in the London Underground asks for money so more research can be done into heart and circulatory diseases. Another advertisement reminds us that everyone will suffer from rheumatism sooner or later and that money spent on research would be the best investment. Others want money for cancer research.

In 1970 President Nixon thought that with enough money cancer would be vanquished during his presidency. He brought together the best American experts, who were all equally convinced that with enough money the victory over cancer would be achieved in a short space of time. Billions of dollars were given to the programme. Ten years later, the same experts met again and could only express their disappointment.

AIDS, which has spread terror in the West in the last few years, has been a good opportunity to reinforce the traditional mental pictures about health. A sentence in a well-respected French newspaper perfectly reflects the prevailing ideas: 'The West suddenly finds itself confronted by a terrible threat which is not due to the madness of men, but to a brutal attack, up to now unstoppable, from a foreign virus which comes from somewhere beyond our world.' Since the AIDS scare began, the big multinational pharmaceutical companies have been poised to devote huge sums of money to market a specific vaccine against AIDS as fast as possible. Yet again, the necessity urgently to solve precise problems does not allow fundamental questions to be explored. Who would dare ask for money to study the genesis of good health?

## The Genesis of Good Health

The starting point for research in primal health is to ask questions about why people are healthy rather than why people are ill. This is poles apart from the conventional approach which only asks questions about why people get a particular disease. Smoking is a good illustration of the huge gulf between the two approaches. The questions usually asked about smoking are: How can you stop smoking? What can you do to break the addiction? What are the best methods for giving up smoking? Is public education helpful? Should cigarettes be modified to make them less dangerous? Should cigarette advertising be banned, or altered? Would the consumption of cigarettes go down if the price went up? And so on.

Research into primal health confronts the root of the problem. Why is it that a great proportion of the population has never felt the need to smoke? What do non-smokers have in common? Such questions would lead us to explore the primal period first.

One could imagine a wealth of research programmes concerned with primal health. There would be a variety of different ways to study adults and old people who met certain criteria of good health. One could research everything there was to know about the conditions of their conception, the lifestyle of their mothers during pregnancy, the way they were born, the way they were fed during infancy, and the social environment during the primal period. Of course, such studies would run into difficulties, particularly when one wanted to study groups of people over fifty years old. Control groups would not be impossible, even if it meant including people who had died. The main practical difficulty would be the imprecise nature of many of the findings. However, such studies would be relatively cheap and would probably reveal some fruitful new information. They would give a particular importance to epidemiology, a discipline which· has a great future. Epidemiology investigates the health of populations. It looks at risk factors for certain diseases, evaluates methods of prevention and often influences the politics of health. It is among epidemiologists that one finds the greatest number of doctors whose awareness comes closest to the concept of primal health.

But the real difficulties are not practical ones. The first difficulty is to find a way of studying the genesis of good health on a global scale instead of concentrating on each particular disease. By ignoring the works of pioneers such as Antoine Béchamp, we lost a whole century. Béchamp, who knew about germs before Pasteur, wrote in support of his theoretical views: 'There are no germs and no bacteria which are intrinsically harmful in order to make men and animals ill. . . . the primary cause of our diseases is inside us, always inside us.'

The second difficulty is more profound. We live in a society dominated by the male, where the model is a masculine one. Such a society devalues those things which are specifically female: pregnancy, childbirth and breast-feeding. Such a society pays no attention to the fetus and the newborn. To be interested in babies and to be interested in the distant future is feminine. The science typical of our society represents the masculine parts of our brain.

Researchers and clinicians have tried to study the process of attachment, the ties between mother and baby, in a scientific way. They are pioneers and have to face many difficulties. Some people think it is ridiculous that serious academics spend time and money proving that a newborn baby needs its mother and that the mother needs her baby. But in a mad society which applauds the most aberrant behaviour, any proof that establishes how solid fundamental human needs are is desirable. However, the time and money spent on researching the bonding process is a drop in the ocean compared with that spent, for example, promoting a new tranquillizer.

The only people who have really tried to establish correlations between the primal period and adulthood are those who have explored the development of learning abilities, intelligence and sensory functions. Why are there so many studies about the beginning of intelligence and about the development of learning abilities? And why are there so few studies about the genesis of health and about the factors which can influence the way a person learns to recognize bacteria, or a virus, or a cancer cell, or learns how to adapt to changes of temperature, or learns how to adjust his hormonal levels or his blood pressure?

Paradoxically, research into primal health seems to be more advanced with plants than with humans. For example, the tolerance of spinach to the cold has been carefully studied; it seems to increase if it experienced low temperatures at the beginning of its life, at the beginning of its growing period.

## Correlations between the Primal Period and Disease

Even if our society is not yet interested in the genesis of good health for human beings, the dawn of a new awareness might at least spark off some new lines of questioning about the factors involved in diseases.

Once you are aware of the importance of the primal period, your curiosity is constantly aroused, no matter what disease is being considered. There are endless examples of this. Take for example people with a high level of cholesterol. The most elementary curiosity would make you ask how these people were fed as infants. It is known that human breast milk has a higher amount of cholesterol than artificial milk. There are reasons to suspect that in order to compensate for the relative deficit, the bottle-fed baby adjusts its synthesis of cholesterol at too high a level. Up to now the only information we have is that there is a greater frequency of atheroma deposits in people aged under twenty who were bottle-fed.

The same basic curiosity would also make us question how patients with gall stones were fed as babies. We know that human breast milk is rich in an amino acid called taurine and that when bile acids mix with taurine the secretion of bile salts and the flow of bile are easier. Babies cannot synthesize taurine easily – they need to have it from breast milk. So the question is whether problems with bile later in life can be traced back to the time when the patient was bottle fed as a baby.

Some facts about leukemia might also stimulate our curiosity in the same way. Leukemia in baby mice – often used as a model for human leukemia – is contracted on the first day of life. We know that leukemia is particularly common in some countries such as Finland, Israel, Sweden and some American states. These are all places where medical technology deeply disturbs the period around birth. So it would be essential to study the conditions of birth itself and the first days of life in patients with leukemia. Until now, the only thing that was looked at in the whole primal period was the place of birth.

As a further example, let us take children (mostly boys) with a variety of symptoms. They are dyslexic; they are often left-handed; they have allergic conditions; they are often especially gifted at mathematics. When the brains of boys such as these have been examined in a post-mortem after an accidental death, it seemed that this set of symptoms corresponds to a late development of nervous cells in the left hemisphere, compared to a faster development in the right hemisphere. Insofar as cerebral dominance is connected with sex hormones, it seems that these characteristics might be associated with particular fluctuations of male hormones during pregnancy. Even if genetic factors are probably involved, it is still tempting to ask what happened during the pregnancies of their mothers.

As a last example, let us look at that very common condition, psoriasis. This is primarily a skin disease charac-

123

terized by red scaly areas that are often itchy. It often starts around puberty, mostly in boys. The condition gets more common the further north you go. People suffering from psoriasis have a very low level of melatonin, the hormone secreted by the pineal gland, especially at night. So psoriasis might be a symptom of a bad adaptation to darkness. Going out into the sun is one of the best ways of bringing about a remission.

Once again, our curiosity drives us back to the beginning of life when the biological clock was being regulated and the activity of the pineal gland adjusted. The question is whether people with psoriasis had enough darkness during the period following birth. This does not exclude the importance of probable genetic factors.

It is certainly possible to find studies which do suggest the importance of the beginning of life in determining certain diseases scattered around the medical literature. But there are very few, and they are about a great many different areas. Generally they have not attracted the attention of the medical profession to any great extent. They are nonetheless often highly significant.

Recently the results of an enquiry were published, which might become a kind of model. A New York team looked into suicide amongst adolescents – a true disease of our civilization. We know that in the last thirty years the rate of adolescent suicide has tripled, while the suicide rate for adults has stayed pretty much the same. Among a group of fifty-two adolescents who committed suicide, with two control groups, the New York team analysed forty-six risk factors which corresponded to the period around birth. The authors of the study found that a large proportion of the adolescent suicides had been resuscitated at birth. Of course, one such study is not enough. But it does pave the way for a type of investigation which will become more and more necessary in the future and which will allow us to establish connections between things never thought of before.

Doctors have been playing the role of the sorcerer's apprentice to such an extent during the second half of this century that only well-programmed computers will be able to unearth and unravel all the nasty surprises lying in wait for future generations. For example, is it unreasonable to imagine that in the middle of the next century we will be able to make connections between the extensive use of ultrasound in obstetrics now and a greater frequency of certain illnesses or characteristics among people who will then be over fifty?

At the moment, such long-term studies are exceptional. They do, however, exist, although they are scattered and their real value is not appreciated. For example, my attention was drawn to a doctor's study of a very common type of vertigo. The author showed that what the majority of patients had in common was the fact that they had not been cuddled and caressed at the beginning of their lives and had hardly ever had tender words spoken to them.

In a similar way, my attention was attracted by a study about excess secretion of prolactin. Some women secrete milk without having given birth to a baby during the previous months, and they also have no periods. The study showed that most of these women had no father at the beginning of their lives, or else that the father was violent and alchoholic. Another enquiry, which can be seen as one of these rare investigations, looked at cancer of the testicles, a disease which is becoming more and more common. This study asked questions about fetal life and about hormonal imbalances which might have disturbed the pregnancy.

Short-term investigations are less exceptional, however. For example, an American study showed that among children who had cancer before the age of four there was a significant number who had weighed more than 4 kg at birth. This suggests the importance of factors which influence fetal life.

A Scottish team studied children aged ten whose birth weight had been less than 2.5 kg to see if there was any connection between various common handicaps and low birth weight. In the category of short-term studies we can include statistics which showed that among abused children, there was a significantly high number of premature babies who had been separated from the mother at birth. Since other statistics have also shown that abused children are more likely than others to become violent adults, the way is open for another study to investigate premature babies separated from their mothers at birth in relation to violence in adulthood.

Niko and Elizabeth Tinbergen were trailblazers in a new generation of research with their work on autistic children. There seem to be more and more autistic children in the industrialized countries. Autistic children avoid all contact with other people, including their mothers; they are not interested in the world around them; they do not talk but often understand spoken language; they do not like changes, and are stuck into routines; they constantly repeat certain movements, such as rocking; they are often hyperactive and have sleep difficulties. By carefully studying each individual history, in particular the beginning of life, the Tinbergens singled out more than twenty factors which applied to autistic children, sometimes finding as many as four, five or more in the same child. These are the things they found with significant frequency:

deep forceps delivery
immediate separation between mother and baby at birth
hospitalization early in life
many journeys, and frequently meeting strangers between the ages of 8 to 30 months
being pushed to achieve things too early

the mother's job, particularly intellectual professions which preoccupied her even when she was at home
the sudden disappearance of a familiar person.

The Tinbergens took the precaution of studying eleven pairs of identical twins so that they could eliminate genetic factors as the primary cause.

Studies in Scandinavia established a relationship between breastfeeding and insulin-dependent diabetes. In the various Scandinavian countries the rate of breastfeeding dropped considerably between 1944 and the end of the 1960s. Then it began to rise again from 1970. It was observed that the level of diabetes rose following the decrease in breastfeeding, beginning to show up nine years later. The number of cases of diabetes dropped following an increase in breastfeeding. These observations led to a study which looked at how hundreds of diabetic children had been fed as infants. It was found that they had been breastfed for a shorter than average time.

The kind of questions asked in studies such as these is much more important than the results or the methods used, and distinguishes such studies from others. The same kind of questions inspired studies whose starting point was quite different. These are the longitudinal studies which follow a population of babies far into their future. Typical of these are three national British studies which respectively began in 1946, 1958 and 1970. They took all the babies born in the same week in the same year and followed them through at regular intervals. Apparently the questions are of most interest to psychologists, psychiatrists and sociologists – even when the information is about asthma, hearing problems or some long-term consequences of smoking during pregnancy. However, these studies are full of promise, particularly the one which started in 1970 and which did include questions and answers about pregnancy and childbirth.

127

Another longitudinal study following children from birth to fifteen years of age was designed to determine the risk of allergies correlated with the food ingested during the first months of life. The results of this study showed that the breastfed infants had the lowest risk of allergic diseases. It also showed that feeding babies with soya milk produced no advantage over cow's milk.

## New Kinds of Research

An even newer kind of study, unimaginable at the present time by people with a conventional outlook, will probably develop in the near future. All the therapists who use powerful regression, in which control by the neocortex is greatly reduced, stress the importance of birth, underlining the long-term consequences of the conditions of birth. This applies to primal therapy, rebirthing, therapies which use hypnosis and therapies which use psychedelic drugs.

From my own practice I learned that there is a correlation between the way a baby girl is born and the way she will give birth to her own children. I also learned that when someone had a difficult birth, there was a tendency for that person to make any birth he or she witnessed difficult as well. Observations such as these might inspire a wealth of research.

Let us imagine, for example, a study to find out about the births of a group of midwives and obstetricians, and then look and see what correlations there were between the rate of forceps, the rate of caesarians, the rate of perinatal deaths in the babies they delivered, and the way they had been born themselves! In the same way, we might do a study which looked at the effects of the presence of the baby's father during a labour, then look at his own birth, and see if any connections could be made.

Let us imagine that we found a way of showing that a

128

doctor's efficiency depended more on his primal state of health than on his knowledge of pharmacology! Such studies might lead to essential practical conclusions at a time when normal childbirth is more and more rare, and when most doctors are poor healers.

These thoughts about the future of research confirm that, contrary to belief, skill and technology are often further ahead than science. The past gives us many examples. The effects of acupuncture or morphine or aspirin were known for a long time before it was understood how they worked. The steam engine was invented before the laws of thermodynamics were known. Vaccinations were used before immunology. The same is true for research in primal health. Because our technological society does so much to disturb the period of dependence on the mother in so many different ways we now urgently need a new awareness, a new way of looking at health and new kinds of research.

# CHAPTER 10

# Primal Health and 'Prise de Conscience'*

Even if we have enough scientific data to understand the importance of primal health, much more than that is in fact needed. What we must have is a new awareness. Such a new awareness could shake up every aspect of our society.

## The Nuclear Family

The nuclear family is one of the most destructive aspects of today's society. It ignores the fundamental needs of a pregnant woman, of a woman in labour and of an infant. In the traditional extended family a woman expecting a baby is always surrounded by women of different generations who help each other in their everyday lives, including the tasks of motherhood. In this sort of extended family, a first-time mother gains experience of newborn babies in advance.

In a nuclear family the pregnant woman either stays at

* See Linguistic note, p. 8.

home with long hours spent alone, or goes out to work and is unable to adapt her lifestyle to the different phases of the pregnancy. In the professional world, if a woman announces that she is pregnant there is a feeling she will be less efficient and less cost-effective. On the day of the birth itself, a mother needs privacy – but she also needs to feel that she is part of a community. These two needs cannot easily be satisfied in our society.

During the months of breastfeeding, the traditional extended family can help the mother-to-be with her baby as much as possible, day and night. If the mother is busy, then another woman in the family is always there to meet the baby's needs. So the baby always has someone's arms at his disposal for the first year of his life, and there is always someone to play with him. In such an arrangement the baby can often be with old people, such as grandparents who have their own special ways with newborn babies. And this contact with babies means that old people have something to live for.

The specific qualities of the mother's role and the father's role tend to be diminished by the nuclear family, by breastfeeding which is short and incomplete and by modern ways of giving birth. No society has ever ignored to such an extent as ours the bipolarity between masculine and feminine which is necessary for the development of a human being. It is impossible at the moment to calculate the long-term consequences of such a new situation.

In our modern industrialized society, everything is constantly conspiring to reduce the size of the family. The birth rate gets lower and lower so that the number of children in a family is less and less. In China, everything is done to discourage a second child – which means the future obliteration of the words brother and sister! Single parents are more and more common in Western societies. Even when family members are not scattered all over the place, fast-changing moral values and attitudes mean that there are often misunderstandings and conflicts inside the family. The rise in the standard of living and modern technology both contribute to the reduction in family size and to make the nuclear family a model. Architects and town planners now design housing that is spread out because nearly everyone has a telephone and a car; indeed, the size of cars perfectly matches the size of the nuclear family. We cannot consider the nuclear family without considering the whole technological society on which it depends.

## Obstetrics

Certain institutions belonging to the technological society have a powerful influence on what happens during the primal period. Of these obstetrics is probably one of the most powerful. Since the priority of obstetrics is to control childbirth, it is likely to defend the concentration of births in big hospitals and the monitoring of women in labour by electronic machinery. In view of this, obstetrics will take no account of factors which could help the physiological process, either in childbirth or in the process of attachment.

Everyone who has tried to understand what makes childbirth easier, less painful, shorter and thus less dangerous is agreed. They all emphasize the importance of a familiar and feminine environment. They know that the presence of a doctor is often inhibiting. They know that when you have to go from one place to another during labour it can often disturb things. And they know how important are semi-darkness, silence, warmth and freedom of position.

When roughly four-fifths of the population of the Western world live less than twenty minutes from a hospital equipped to do caesarians; when even ambulances for dogs have the equipment needed to do emergency surgery, there can be no rational basis for the discredit accorded to home

132

birth. This discredit is based on a lack of will. The subtlest way to discredit home birth is to make it as dangerous as possible. It is made dangerous partly by creating an atmosphere of guilt. When a woman dares to think of having a home birth, the first thing she is asked is what she would do if there were complications. Professionals never think that it might be easier if women did not have to leave a familiar place. Home birth is made dangerous by maintaining an atmosphere of conflict. When a midwife has to transfer a labouring woman from home to hospital, she knows she is open to criticism and even to ridicule. Home birth is also made dangerous because there is no training for authentic midwives, and the women who could do the best job are not the ones who are selected. Age (old enough to have had her own children), experience, initiative and the ability to make her own decisions are the principal qualities needed in a midwife working with home births.

With the training of midwives as it is at the moment, not only are we not getting authentic midwives, but we are often stopping the careers at an early stage of those women who genuinely want to help other women give birth. This is done either by hassles with authority, or because it is hard to earn your living this way. These tangles with authority are usually subtle and hard to pinpoint. They also involve the rare doctors who do home births. These doctors are often attacked indirectly for their 'incompetence', their 'faults' outside the field of childbirth. Economic pressures also have various ways of being felt. In France the amount reimbursed by the social security to a mother having a home birth is hardly enough to pay for the midwife. In the USA, the decision by some big insurance companies (Mutual Fire Marine and Inland Insurance Company of Philadelphia) not to cover private 'nurse-midwives' for home births is an efficient and discreet model of repression by economic means.

There is an area in which there has been no progress in the last thirty years. This is the study of factors which can influence the hormonal balance necessary for childbirth, either in a positive or a negative way. This subject is taboo and subversive; it would lead to the basis of obstetrics being reconsidered. It would lead to the total reconsideration of certain practices which are performed every day. Such practices include women in labour having to leave their house, travelling in a car or ambulance, undergoing a number of vaginal examinations and having a needle inserted in a vein – all within a few hours. All these are ways, hitherto unsuspected, of blocking the physiological process of childbirth.

If obstetrics had the slightest interest in the physiology of childbirth, some routines would be reconsidered, criticized, discussed and used discerningly. Let us take as a simple example the practice of putting a drip in the arm of a labouring woman. No one has ever proved that the effects of adrenalin secreted when a needle is inserted are negligible. Moreover, it is uncommon to be interested in the undesirable effects of glucose in the drip. Yet it has been discovered only very recently that glucose received in a drip can actually increase sensitivity to pain. Glucose also lowers the level of sodium chloride in the blood of both mother and baby. A low level of sodium chloride in the baby has the effect of making it breathe too fast. There is also evidence that a high level of glucose blocks the synthesis of prostaglandins, whose role is so important during childbirth. The baby reacts to the excess of sugar by activating its pancreas and secreting more insulin. The result is that after the birth the newborn baby is hypoglycemic. This might help explain the increase in neonatal jaundice in the last ten years. It is also significant that when a labouring woman has no drug and is absolutely free to drink what she wants, she often only wants water. If she chooses to drink something sweet, it is often because she has been told she needs to boost her energy.

It is because it takes no account of physiology that obstetrics is dangerous. To keep the mortality rate down to around ten per thousand, the caesarian rate must often reach 20 per cent and the rate of forceps 30 per cent for a first baby. The number of women who succeed in giving birth to their first baby without the use of drugs and using only their own hormones is getting less and less. In many modern hospitals more than 10 per cent of newborn babies are under the surveillance of pediatricians rather than the mother for the first few days of the baby's life. This is often because of the effect of drugs on the baby during childbirth. In contrast, wherever experienced midwives are autonomous and have at their disposal a surgical team who could do a caesarian at any time in a properly equipped theatre, the perinatal mortality rate can be around ten per thousand and the caesarian rate below 10 per cent. Under these conditions, there are the lowest possible risks to the mother and never any need to recourse to drugs.

It would thus be possible to improve considerably the safety of birth both in the long and short term by adopting an approach which is radically different from, and incompatible with, the absolute control exercised by the institution of medicine. Instead of the present state of affairs, one must imagine doctors and techniques which would be at the service of women and midwives; one must imagine doctors who are capable of studying the physiological processes with the aim of helping them, and not with the ulterior motive of controlling them.

What I say must not be taken as a criticism of obstetricians. The majority of obstetricians, taken individually, are people of good faith whose main concern is that as many babies as possible are born in good health. My criticisms are directed more against the institution of obstetrics. Beyond a certain size, the priority of any institution is to maintain its identity rather than to be interested in society as a whole. Society is in the process of losing control over some of its institutions. My criticisms must not be taken either to suggest that I envisage home birth as the only possible alternative to obstetrics. The essential thing is to rediscover the role of authentic midwives, who are the only people who do not disturb the physiology of childbirth.

The role played by obstetrics in the evolution of family and social structures is probably much more important than is normally supposed. Birth is the key event which traditionally separated the world of men and the world of women. The relationship between men and women in a birthing place does more than just reflect society as a whole: it plays a determinant role in the maintenance and evolution of family structures. It is not by chance that in the middle of the twentieth century women suddenly needed to be assisted by the baby's father during childbirth and even to share the experience with him. Before this time, either the father was excluded, as he had been in most traditional societies, or his presence was tolerated and justified by his performing practical tasks, like filling up basins of water.

This unprecedented sociological phenomenon has coincided with the concentration of births in hospital and with the evolution of the nuclear family. It has also coincided with a decline in the role of the midwife. This decline has taken different forms in different countries. But, no matter what term is used to describe it, the fact is that the midwives who have survived have become auxiliaries of doctors. Nowadays it is not possible to define the midwife's job without referring to the medical profession. Either the midwife is officially considered as an auxiliary to a doctor, or else her job is considered as a medical profession with limited competence. Midwives are less and less autonomous. There are fewer and fewer authentic midwives.

Nowadays, in most Western countries, the presence of

the father at the birth has become a rule, accepted by even the most conservative maternity wards. The presence of the father reinforces the image of the nuclear family as the model, just as the nuclear family reinforces the image of the father at birth as the model. It is obvious that the presence of the baby's father has become a necessity in the context of modern obstetrics. It is also part of a trend to make hospitals more human. But do men really have a place in circumstances where the priorities would be different; in circumstances where women would be able to give birth using their own hormones? The part fathers play in sharing emotions is rarely questioned. Is it always positive? To dare ask such a question is almost scandalous at a time when childbirth is thought of as something just between a couple. But, having observed thousands of couples, who come from every kind of socio-economic group, it seems that things are not so simple as people think. The kind of bond between couples and the kind of intimacy they share can be incredibly different. The anxiety which fathers feel about birth is very different from one man to another.

I have a feeling that men who had an easy birth themselves usually play a positive role in childbirth, and vice versa. Some fathers disguise their anxiety by being very active and by talking a lot. An anxious man wants to massage his wife and to control her breathing and her position. He tends to be possessive. There are sometimes latent conflicts going on inside couples and this can come out in a birth which is long and difficult. Many men, because they are men, are surprised and disturbed by the internal trip a woman makes to bring a child into the world.

The behaviour of some men during childbirth is perhaps more akin to the behaviour of primitive men. Men like this often play a positive role. They keep themselves in the background, sometimes even outside the room, as if to protect the privacy of their childbearing wives from the world outside. Perhaps behaviour like this is not very different from how it used to be in the primitive societies of hunter-gatherers: the men kept guard, protecting their women from the outside world and protecting the birth of their babies. Certainly, it is not very different from some animals. For example, when a baby dolphin is being born, the males stay outside the group of females, always at the ready to kill sharks.

The father's common participation has largely contributed to the role of the midwife being reduced nowadays to one of technique. I am constantly reminded in daily practice of the irreplaceable role of an experienced midwife. Let me give an example. A labour is long, and does not seem to be progressing. The dilation of the cervix stays the same for several hours. The father then decides to leave the room for a short while. During his short absence, the baby is born. Because of the father's new role, it is easy to forget how positive women can be – women such as the mother or sister of the labouring woman – as long as they gave birth by themselves, meaning without medical intervention.

A woman in labour needs to have a special relationship with one other person. Sometimes this means that she has to make a choice, because if there are several people present at the birth it can be counterproductive. I sometimes say that the length of the labour is in direct proportion to the number of people present!

## The World of Men and the World of Women

Why is it that for thousands of years women in labour have always hidden away from mens' eyes while they gave birth? No doubt they felt that their need for privacy would have been disturbed by the presence of men. Apparently the traditional needs of a woman giving birth are not the same as women of today.

138

We must remember that in traditional societies women shared their daily lives, and shared intimate things with each other, such as when they were having a period. So when a woman gave birth, the presence of other women with whom she was already intimate was not felt as a disturbance. In contrast, some Western women can only find privacy in the bathroom. But the differences between these two groups of women are only superficial. What they share is a common need for privacy. Even if modern couples share a kind of intimacy that was unknown before modern Western society, it is still probable that the consequences of men looking on during childbirth is not so very different now.

There are some things which a labouring woman does which she would not usually do in front of her sexual partner. For example, during childbirth a woman needs to empty her rectum. This is rather something she might feel comfortable doing in front of her mother. The kind of privacy which a labouring woman needs is not disturbed by the presence of an authentic midwife, someone who is a motherly woman as well as an experienced one.

Privacy is indeed the key word in an understanding of the needs of a woman giving birth. Privacy is what you feel when there is no social control. It goes with a reduction in control by the neocortex, the upper brain. The active part of the brain during childbirth is the archaic brain, the primal brain; the brain we have in common with all the other mammals. It is the primal brain which secretes all the hormones necessary for childbirth. Childbirth is an involuntary process, but this involuntary process can be disturbed by the activity of the neocortex. All inhibitions come from the neocortex. Helping a woman give birth means helping her reduce the control of the neocortex, or not doing things to prevent this. It means not preventing her from cutting herself off from the outside world. Men have never been able to make the interior trip of childbirth, and that is why many of them can disturb things by their presence. Obstetrics, a medical discipline which is dominated by male doctors, has never understood the physiology of childbirth.

Another reason why it might be necessary to keep the worlds of men and women separate is to maintain sexual attraction. Sexual attraction needs an element of mystery. At the time when men were hunter-gatherers the birth of a baby in the world of women was shrouded in mystery. Goddesses were worshipped. In the same sort of way it is possible that certain aspects of the mens' world, such as hunting, fired the fantasies of women. Nowadays, in our unisex society where there is little distinction between men and women, the element of mystery has almost gone. I have been taken aback by the large number of divorces and separations among couples who shared marvellous birth experiences. On the other hand, couples where the man was not an active participant in the birth of his children seem to still have solid relationships.

The interest which a man has in a newborn baby follows a kind of chronology; it gets stronger as the baby gets older. This is not the same for a woman, who has what is called 'the primary maternal preoccupation', which is connected with profound biological changes. Perhaps there is a tendency nowadays to upset this paternal chronology. Not only are the positive effects of the father sharing the birth now accepted without discussion, but some people actually teach the father to touch the baby inside the mother's tummy – without waiting for him to do it spontaneously. Perhaps the main role of the father should be to protect and help the mother/baby couple, to satisfy their needs, before he establishes a direct attachment with the baby.

What I have said does not mean there is no place for the father in the birthing room. His presence is often felt to be necessary in the context of the nuclear family and of hospital confinements. But it is appropriate to ask why the world of women was traditionally protected from men's sight.

For their part, men have always sought ways to give more importance to themselves in the period around childbirth. This tendency has expressed itself differently according to the different stages of history – or, more precisely, according to the different stages in the history of patriarchy. The rite of the *couvade* seems to correspond to the first stage, with the passage from matriarchy to patriarchy. *Couvade* is when the man does various things to imitate a woman giving birth. The man goes to bed, expresses pain and stops his social activities in a ritualistic way. He does this in such a way that other people devote their care to him, and offer him their congratulations. It is sometimes the man who introduces the new baby to the community. The phenomenon of the *couvade*, with local variations, was known to Herodotus amongst African tribes, by Nymphodorus amongst the Scythians of the Black Sea, by Diodorus in Corsica, by Strabo amongst the ancestors of the Basques and by Marco Polo amongst the mountain tribes of Miau-tse. Today the *couvade* can still be found in places which are far apart from each other, such as Siberia, South America, Africa and Malaysia.

With the arrival of monotheistic religions, the power of men over women during the period around birth took on new forms. The Christian baptism could be interpreted as the true birth, the spiritual birth given by the religious fathers. Women are reduced to only being able to give birth biologically. Circumcision in the first eight days of life can be interpreted as the penetration by man in the world of women. Only men could originate such a cruel custom. Mothers left to themselves would be very unlikely to do that to their own baby boys.

But, of course, it is through the medical institution that men have taken control of childbirth most powerfully. The doctor has weakened the role of the midwife by creating a

141

professional whose education he controlled. Not only has medicine increased its control over childbirth itself, but during the twentieth century it has also wanted to teach women how to give birth. Lamaze wrote that a woman must learn how to give birth in the same way that one learns how to swim, read or write! This attitude has done a lot to contribute to the profound misunderstanding of the physiology of birth.

Today the common participation of the father seems to be the next stage in the masculinization of the birth place, and of the feminization of man. Although most antenatal teachers and childbirth educators are women, some of what they teach comes from male obstetricians. Some teachers even promote a method whereby the man is instructed how to coach his wife during labour and delivery. This kind of attitude has largely contributed to people holding on to the idea that a delivery can be actively helped, whereas the essential reality is that above all else a delivery should not be disturbed.

One must not forget the other stage in the masculinization of childbirth – the male midwife. It is now possible for a woman giving birth to be surrounded by three men: the male midwife, the baby's father and the doctor. Under such conditions, a woman rarely gives birth by herself. Even if she escapes a caesarian, her uterus cannot be considered to do its job properly without the help of artificial hormones, carefully administered by the professionals. All the mystery has gone. There are no more goddesses any longer.

We have reached such a degree of absurdity that two questions immediately need to be asked: What chances of survival has a society got without midwives? In other words, a society which completely denies the complementary roles of males and females. Second, is a new awareness still possible? I prefer to answer just the second question and express my optimism. All over the world, mothers feel called towards the vocation of midwifery after having had their own children. They rediscover the true role of the midwife. More and more women are searching for alternatives to conventional obstetrical birth. There are professionals who do things which are outside the law so they can abide by the body's physiological processes. Medico-legal institutions need to use more and more force to put a brake on this movement. Some midwives have been in prison. Some doctors have been disqualified because their attitude was considered 'bizarre'. There would not have been such witchhunts in various countries if this movement had just been a passing fashion. Obstetrics is the medical discipline which has contributed most to the weakening of primal health in our society.

## Neonatology

The effects of obstetrics are powerfully reinforced by the up and coming discipline of neonatology – the medicine of newborn babies. The Frenchman Pierre Budin may be considered as the first neonatologist. Pierre Budin knew that one must not separate mother and baby. Paradoxically though, it was his pupil Martin Cooley who created the first 'nursery' in 1896 and imposed complete separation between the premature baby and its mother. Nowadays the symbol of neonatology is the incubator.

An incubator is nothing more than a glass box with a thermostat. Until now, the criticisms of the incubator have always been directed against some particular aspects of the incubator rather than against the whole concept. For example, some people thought that when the baby was in an incubator he was not able to move enough, so his vestibular system was not stimulated enough. This might explain why the baby stopped breathing in certain cases. So the oscillating bed was invented. Other people thought the

143

baby was not getting enough skin stimulation. So they invented TLC – tender loving care. This meant that at regular times, according to a timetable, a dutiful nurse would come and stroke the baby's skin. Others drew attention to the fact that the baby inside an incubator could only hear the sound of the machinery, so they thought of introducing a recording of the mother's voice. Some thought of putting a towel into the incubator which had the mother's smell on it, knowing that the sense of smell plays an important role in the identification of the mother by the baby. Others were primarily concerned about the bacterial environment in an incubator, which was different from the bacterial environment around the mother. Still others emphasized that when a mother is separated from her baby she has difficulty in secreting milk.

A few people have dared to reconsider the incubator itself. A team in Bogota, Colombia, has gone the furthest. They were inspired by marsupials: the baby kangaroo is born long before it is mature, and is kept in a pouch next to its mother's skin and mammary glands. The Bogota team has shown that the human mother can be the best incubator. The 'kangaroo method' consists of keeping the baby in contact with its mother's skin day and night, in a vertical position, with the mother's clothes acting as a pouch. This is not considered possible unless the baby's lungs are mature, which means the baby does not need artificial respiration. Mother and baby can also go straight back home, to the bacterial environment where the baby is going to be living. If the baby needs any supplementary feeding this is never given in the form of artificial milk, but as guava juice. After only a short time, the results from this approach are already impressive. For babies weighing less than 1 kg at birth the survival rate went up from 0 per cent to 72 per cent. For babies weighing between 1 kg and 1.5 kg the rate went up from 27 per cent to 89 per cent.

There are some who say that the Bogota team does not

have any statistician and that some babies who are stillborn or who die immediately after birth are not taken into account. Others think that their approach is only appropriate for third world countries (which means two-thirds of humanity!). It is obvious that the last people to understand the true nature of the revolution in Bogota are neonatologists, who will fight to the end to preserve the symbol of their own discipline – the incubator. It is also obvious that no compromise is possible between the Bogota approach and the context of an intensive care unit. One has to make a choice; or, rather, a big leap. It is too early to evaluate the long-term implications of the Bogota approach, but already they can say that the number of babies who are hospitalized later is considerably reduced. It is also possible that the 'kangaroo method' will have a good effect on the rate of juvenile delinquency, which is a problem in Bogota.

The Bogota approach is radically different from the conventional medical one. First, it involves exploiting to the full the physiological human potential, before looking for a substitute. Second, it has a long-term vision, which goes beyond taking only survival rates into account.

The concept of primal health is not just about new mental pictures. It involves a total new awareness, a new light in the dark. At the moment there are only a few scattered glimmers of this light, such as the one bright torch of Bogota.

# CHAPTER 11

# Windows on the Future

Our critique of the nuclear family and of institutions like obstetrics and neonatology will remind many of that famous island Utopia. But health does have a place in Utopia. Health is a struggle, a constant and never-ending effort towards perfect adaptation. To be realistic we first of all have to admit that our technological society cannot survive without undergoing an enormous mutation. However, we need the concept of Utopia; we need goals to aim for. It is obvious that it needs time to change family structures, and it is also obvious that a network of authentic midwives cannot be organized overnight.

When a whole way of life is challenged, from birth to death, it needs time. One cannot disassociate the possible ways of rediscovering the extended family from how people are born and how they die. Unless a large proportion of the population can choose to give birth at home and die at home, family structures will never be enlarged. This means adopting another attitude towards medicine; it means a new understanding of the dangers of hospital-centred medicine. Many people in our society die in hospitals, simply because hospitals are now considered the normal place to die. People who die in hospitals are often subjected to painful

146

interventions, and suffer in a futile way. We have to rediscover the art of birthing and the art of dying in parallel.

Even so, a new awareness of the concept of primal health can have almost immediate practical effects. For example, what is there to stop most mothers from moving around with their baby in a baby carrier? In traditional societies, most babies spent a great part of their waking hours close to their mother's body, on her hip or in a sling, or held by someone else.

On the walls of the maternity unit at Pithiviers we display a whole collection of pictures showing babies being carried in a variety of different carriers, in many different cultures. When you consider how much stimulation a baby is aware of, you see that there is no comparison between the constant contact with the mother's body which a baby gets in a baby carrier and the lack of body contact when a baby is lying in a pram. It was only in the 1960s and 1970s that the baby carrier was rediscovered in the Western world. Everyone who has used a carrier knows how effective it is in pacifying and reassuring a baby. For the baby, it is another way to discover the world.

Also, nothing should prevent all babies from sleeping with their mothers. This does not involve any expense, it does not need any equipment and it falls outside the control of the big institutions. In every society, with the notable exception of Western society since the eighteenth century, babies always slept with their mothers. It takes only the most elementary observation to see that a baby needs its mother even more during the night than during the day, and even more in the dark than in the daylight. In the dark the baby's predominant sense – sight – is at rest. Instead, the baby needs to use its sense of touch through skin-to-skin contact, and its sense of smell.

The mother needs the baby too. Anyone who knows about difficulties with breastfeeding in our society knows that one of the main explanations for this is that babies are separated from their mothers at night. Also, many young mothers have sleeping difficulties because they are separated from their babies. In a maternity unit where mothers are allowed to give birth using their own hormones, in an atmosphere which gives them the freedom to be spontaneous, many tend to sleep with their babies and carry on doing so once they return home.

If mothers do not sleep with their babies, it is because someone has told them it is a bad habit. For the last three centuries, women have been told this, first in the name of morality, and then in the name of science. Mothers of previous generations like to respect what they themselves were taught. What they call 'bad habits' are in fact normal and natural ways of meeting a baby's fundamental needs. Being accused of 'bad habits' is something which can frighten young mothers who would like to listen to their instincts. People warn them that there is a risk of smothering the baby at night, but this simply does not happen; mothers always seem to be aware of their babies even while they are asleep. It is also known that breastfeeding mothers have a particular sleep pattern which excludes the deepest sleep (stage 4). Moreover, a baby in good health knows how to protect himself and raise the alarm if he is bothered by a sheet or blanket over him.

All the women who sleep with their babies say how easy it is to give the breast during the night without waking up completely. They know how the baby uses its sense of smell to find her nipple. The education of the sense of smell is commonly neglected in our society. It is a very archaic function and has a vital role to play in sexual life.

We will never be able to evaluate fully the harmful effects of separating mother and baby at night. For example, SIDS (Sudden Infant Death Syndrome) is becoming increasingly common in Western countries. However, it is difficult to know to what extent habits such as the separation of mother and baby might be responsible. While I was on a visit to

China, I noticed that mothers slept with their babies for at least one year. At the same time, I observed that nobody seemed to understand the meaning of the question when I asked them about 'sudden infant death'. In some countries this is known as 'cot death'. Possibly it is the cot which is the essential factor! Moreover, when you consider how frequent sleeping problems are amongst adults, it is tempting to make a possible connection with the collective habit of disturbing the night-time needs of babies.

Nor can we assess fully the long-term effects of disturbances in breastfeeding which are linked to the common Western habit of separating mother and baby at night. It is also impossible to predict the consequences of all those repeated situations of helplessness and hopelessness brought about by separating mother and baby at night. Separate sleeping is so ingrained in our culture that it is difficult even to talk about them without being laughed at. To change such an apparently simple practice would in fact need very strong social support. And social support is needed even more when dealing with an institution. That is why antenatal teachers and breastfeeding counsellors play such an important role in our society.


## Primal Health Centres

Pregnant women and young mothers need to help each other. They need to have places to meet each other. That is why I plan to set up primal health centres as a first step towards my vision of primal health for everyone. These health centres would act as substitutes for the extended family. Such centres would be places where women and couples thinking of having a baby, pregnant women, young mothers, babies and grandmothers can all get together. It would also be an ideal place for the education of young girls and teenagers; outside our own society, there is not

149

one example where girls can reach the age of motherhood without having held a baby in their arms or ever having seen a newborn baby. Neither the nuclear family nor the school can give this kind of education. Would it not be possible to imagine an arrangement between primal health centres and schools?

A primal health centre would be inseparable from a home birth network, and it could even be a birthing place for some women. Authentic midwives would learn from experience those things which are not known in modern obstetrical units. When I talk about 'authentic midwives' I think of experienced birthing attendants who can recognize the stage of labour without repeating vaginal exams, just by listening to the noise a labouring woman is making, by her posture and by observing the expression on her face.

In the primal health centres I imagine activities to foster a sense of community and group cohesion. None of these activities would be compulsory. For example, there would be discussion groups, singing groups, dancing groups and all sorts of other activities. I imagine a kitchen which would always be open to everybody – a place to learn how to make bread, or how to avoid processed food. Such a kitchen could be the source of the best recipes for a pregnant woman or a breastfeeding mother. A kitchen is somewhere that people immediately feel at ease in, as if they were at home. Such a centre would be a success the day when nobody felt like a guest.

In a place like this it would be possible to develop an unbroken relationship with the childbirth educators, the midwives, the breastfeeding counsellors, and to smash the barriers between professionals and lay people. Dividing lines between everybody's competence and skills would tend to fade with time.

In my dream, many cities would have a primal health centre located near a hospital. But this centre would be careful to preserve its independence vis-à-vis the medical institution. It needs to be kept in mind that medicine plays only a secondary role in the health of a population, and it would only be able to collaborate with a primal health programme in the most discreet way.

There might also be an aquatic feel about the place. Many pregnant women, many mothers and most babies are attracted to water. Small swimming pools might also be used during childbirth to help women release their inhibitions. And babies would be able to cultivate their extraordinary abilities in water. Water makes people dream. And the presence of newborn babies would help people see things more clearly and give them long-term vision. With water and babies, all the conditions are present to create fantasies about the future. It would make these primal health centres windows on the future.

Technology will threaten the survival of humanity as long as it is used by those who cannot develop and exploit their capacity to see into the future. I dream of places which would play a pivotal role in the process of evolution towards a new age. Only healthy people can be conscious of the long-term consequences of their actions and decisions; only healthy people can tackle the real priorities.

I dream that the atmosphere in a primal health centre would be catalytic for discussions about new economics. Imagine economics where the priority is health! What a leap forward in the history of human societies.

I dream that the atmosphere in a primal health centre would be catalytic for radically new ideas about progress. Technological advances will lead to a deathly imbalance unless at the same time man seeks to exploit his archaic brain to its fullest potential. It is his primal brain which determines his state of health and which carries with it another vision of the universe. The destruction of our planet which we are now witnessing can only be the work of a sick man. The priority now is the genesis of a new

151

kind of man, a man who will have another kind of relationship with the Earth, the Mother.

The twenty-first century will be ecological, or will not be.

# Pasteur, An Adventurer in Well-Charted Territory?

My study of primal health led me towards Pasteur and made me understand to what extent Pasteur and his fans solidified the mental pictures associated with the words health and disease. In a completely unforeseen way, I became involved in the 'Pasteur phenomenon', and came across some little-known aspects of his personality and career.

Historians have always viewed Pasteur's career as an enigma. How was it that Pasteur started with crystallography and ended up with vaccination against rabies? Why did Pasteur constantly change the subject of his studies? Why did Pasteur never continue doing basic research in the field in which he had just had some success, switching to another subject instead?

The enigma of his career inspired the author of a recent book to create a diagram illustrating Pasteur's practice of side-stepping. By taking several steps sideways, Pasteur was able to keep an ever-increasing public interested in what he was doing. Thus Pasteur, who had only been of interest to a handful of learned people when he studied crystallography, ended up by being of interest to the whole world when he became involved with vaccination.

Historians of Pasteur would not have met with the same difficulties if they had known about the existence of Antoine Béchamp and the importance of his work. Everything becomes clear when the careers of Pasteur and Béchamp are studied in parallel.

Just a few facts are enough. These facts are irrefutable, and are backed up by documents which can be found in large scientific libraries throughout the world. Today it is possible to claim that Béchamp often preceded Pasteur, and went beyond him; that Pasteur was always aware of the work Béchamp was doing; that Pasteur always gave the impression that he knew nothing about Béchamp; and that Pasteur suppressed and falsified Béchamp's work.

In 1850 Béchamp was professor at the school of pharmacy in Strasbourg. It was in 1854 that Béchamp demonstrated that fermentation is due to microscopic living organisms carried in the air. His conclusions were published on 19 February 1855, at the Academy of Sciences, where he made the following proposition: 'Cold water can only change cane sugar if mould can develop, these elementary fungi acting as fermentation agents.' In 1854 it was impossible that Pasteur was not aware of Béchamp. At that time Pasteur was professor of chemistry at the faculty of sciences in the same city. What is more, in 1854 Béchamp covered for Pasteur while the latter was away in Paris, officially because of a heart condition but in fact to find prestigious supporters to back his promotion.

By 1 August 1854 Pasteur was sufficiently recovered to supervise the examinations, and to receive the six hundred francs due to the examiner. Immediately afterwards Pasteur left for Lille, where he became dean and professor of the new faculty of sciences. He then became interested in fermentation. In 1857, Pasteur published his work on the subject – without even mentioning Béchamp.

The study of diseases of the silk worm is even more significant. At the end of 1854 Béchamp became professor of chemistry and pharmacy at the University of Montpellier. On his own initiative, without any backing and without any financial help, he undertook research on the two diseases affecting silk worms – 'flaccidity' and 'pebrine'. The economic consequences of these diseases were of great importance to the region. In the spring of 1865, Béchamp made a report to the regional agricultural department about the parasitic nature of pebrine and what needed to be done to keep the silk worms healthy. On 20 May 1867 Béchamp reported his conclusions about flaccidity to the Academy of Sciences and demonstrated that the causative agent was a microscopic parasite which he called 'mycrozymas bombycis'. This was the first infection by micro-organisms ever to be described. It was reported in the local newspaper, *Le Messager Du Midi* on 22 May 1867.

In June 1865 Pasteur had left for Alais to study silk worm diseases. At that time he knew nothing about them. On 29 May 1867 – without mentioning Béchamp by name – he ridiculed his research into pebrine: 'Its essential character is precisely in its constitution . . . what an audacious lie it is to say that these microscopic things are outside the eggs and the worms. I think those people are crazy . . .'

Yet by 1868 Pasteur could see that Béchamp had been right. He then set about writing to everybody of any significance (ministers, academics, etc.) saying that he had discovered the parasitic origin of pebrine, and that flaccidity was an independent illness, 'a fact of great importance and entirely unknown before my research.' In 1870 Pasteur published a book about silk worm diseases. The book was dedicated to the Empress Eugenie. Of course, Béchamp is not quoted. Pasteur was invited to Compiègne to the imperial court. He arrived at the sumptuous reception with a microscope and showed the red cells of the Empress to the invited guests. Around this time Pasteur was talking about the cowardice and fanaticism of the republicans.

Some years later, however, after the end of the empire, Pasteur made friends with some freemasons and anti-religious republicans. Thanks to them, he was given a personal income of 12,000 francs a year. This national reward was given to him for saving the silk worm industry.

During the 1880s Béchamp was dean of the Catholic University of Lille. He was beginning to be a threat to Pasteur, daring to pronounce in various scientific reports that he had been frequently ahead of Pasteur in his discoveries. Béchamp decided to publish all his research. As if by chance, in 1888 Béchamp was forced to retire, accused of teaching a materialistic theory. It must not be forgotten that Pasteur had been professor at Lille and still had good friends there.

Of course, Béchamp was not Pasteur's only victim. The Pasteur/Béchamp relationship is just a way of illustrating a radically new theory to explain Pasteur's zig-zag career.

In a similar sort of way, Casimir Davaine was also a victim of Pasteur. Davaine created a methodology to demonstrate that anthrax, a disease affecting both animals and humans, was caused by microbes. Pasteur took the credit for it himself and everybody forgot about Davaine. Then, Pasteur took the credit for finding a vaccination against anthrax which had in fact already been perfectly understood and put to the test by Toussaint before 1880. Pasteur pirated the subject, had some experiments done very fast, compared the safety of Toussaint's vaccine unfavourably with his own, and publicly and triumphantly demonstrated his own procedure – by using Toussaint's vaccine!

Pierre Victor Galtier, professor of the veterinary school in Lyon, had firmly established the theoretical and experimental basis for vaccination against rabies as early as 1879.

Pasteur visited this veterinary college in 1881 accompanied by a student of Galtier. In 1885 Pasteur delivered a presentation to the Academy of Sciences, and the next day to the Academy of Medicine, about his unique trial on vaccination against rabies. What glory! The famous academician Vulpian proclaimed that there had been nobody before Pasteur except Pasteur himself in this field. Pasteur did not contradict this.

The way Pasteur appropriated the works of others is only of historical and anecdotal interest. From a purely practical viewpoint, does it matter whether fermentation and silk worm diseases were understood first by Béchamp, that the role of microbes in some diseases was understood first by Davaine, or that Toussaint and Galtier had been successful in a vaccine against rabies before Pasteur?

In fact, the negative aspect of Pasteur's work is on a much larger scale than this and has to do with something completely different. Indeed, it still affects us today. What is important is the image of illness which, thanks to Pasteur's fame and glory, was taken up and widely spread. In Pasteur's wake medicine looked for an immediate solution to all diseases. Pasteur stifled the voice of all his contemporaries who were asking fundamental questions about *le terrain* and the genesis of good health. This is how Pasteur's glory channelled the hygienist movement, partly eclipsed the work of Claude Bernard and reduced to nothing the work of Béchamp. There were huge consequences for research, for the training of doctors, for medical practice and for the attitude of the general public towards health and disease. In fact, ideas which were put forward by Pasteur at the end of his life have recently been given a new airing. In the end, he would have admitted that 'the microbe is nothing; *le terrain* is everything'.

Pasteur's influence came from his glory, and glory-seeking is the key to the enigma which historians have been unable to resolve until now.

# Glossary

**ACTH (adrenocorticotrophin hormone or corticotrophin)**
This hormone is secreted by the anterior pituitary gland. It controls the output of hormones by the cortex of the adrenal gland, especially cortisol.

ACTH output is in turn controlled by the hypothalamus by means of a complex feedback mechanism which adjusts the body's level of cortisol. For example, if the blood level of cortisol is too high, the output of hypothalamic hormones falls, the output of ACTH falls and the blood level of cortisol drops.

This feedback mechanism has a long latent period: a sudden increase in the level of cortisol, for instance, needs two hours before the secretion of ACTH is inhibited.

**Adrenalin and Noradrenalin**
Both are transmitters of nerve impulses and at the same time are hormones which circulate around the body. They are secreted by the endings of sympathetic nerves and by the adrenal medulla. Belonging to a kind of emergency system, they cause acceleration of the heart, constriction of small blood vessels and an increase in metabolic rate. A

158

surge of adrenalin sends blood rushing to the brain and the muscles to enable a person to fight or run away fast. This blood is drawn from the digestive tract, the uterus and other visceral functions.


## Cortisol

Secreted by the adrenal cortex, this hormone plays a key role in the process of adaptation. It is essential for the normal excretion of water by the kidneys. It tends to cause loss of calcium and phosphates; it raises the blood glucose level; it inhibits the synthesis of proteins; it is a blocking agent in the metabolic pathway of unsaturated fatty acids, and therefore in the synthesis of prostaglandins.

Cortisol plays an important role in the control of blood pressure; it also inhibits the inflammatory process. In situations of helplessness and hopelessness a high level of cortisol is maintained. Depressed people also have a high level. The level at which cortisol has been set at the beginning of life is a key factor in the concept of primal health.


## DNA (deoxyribonucleic acid)

DNA carries the genetic code, which makes each one of us unique.

It determines whether a person will have, for example, brown or blue eyes, dark or brown hair. The chances of two people having the same DNA are infinitesimal.

DNA is capable of making an exact duplicate of itself; it is the key to life. Found primarily in cell nuclei, it has the capacity to manufacture every protein the body can make. So DNA acts as a kind of architect. All cells of the same person have the same DNA, but cells of the different organs become specialized so that only certain genes function. DNA can now be used in new techniques of identification.

## Fatty Acids

1 They are acids which make fats when combined with glycerol.

2 They come from food.

3 The way we metabolize fatty acids represents our state of health in the following ways:

many of the chemical messengers of the body are made from fats (hormones, prostaglandins);
a large proportion of the nervous system is made from fats;
there is an association between the metabolism of minerals and fats;
fatty acids play an important role in all cell membranes and immunity.

4 A fatty acid is a long chain of carbon atoms which ends like any other acid molecule so that it can always combine with an alcohol. Some fatty acids have one or several double bonds. Where there is a double bond a carbon atom can create a further bonding with a hydrogen atom. The fatty acids which can take more hydrogen atoms are called either monounsaturated or polyunsaturated according to the number of double bonds.

5 We need polyunsaturated fatty acids in our diet. Some of them are essential fatty acids, so called because the body needs them and cannot produce them itself. Only two of them are really important: linoleic acid, which is found mostly in seeds, and linolenic acid, which is found mostly in leaves and fish. Our intake of unsaturated fatty acids is usually in the form of vegetable seed oils and fish oils, and offal. Polyunsaturated fatty acids lose their qualities when they are processed or heated at high temperatures. Then they behave like saturated fatty acids.

6 The metabolic pathway of the unsaturated fatty acids needs catalysts (vitamins and minerals). There are also physiological blocking agents (cortisol secreted by the adrenal gland).

**GLA (gamma linolenic acid)**
Precursor of prostaglandins 1, it is a derivative of linoleic acid. It represents an important metabolic crossroad in the maintenance of the function of the T lymphocytes. It modulates the ratio between the different kinds of prostaglandins and has a tendency to favour series 1 over series 2.

Normally the body synthesizes GLA from linoleic acid contained in the diet. However, the synthesis of GLA is commonly disturbed in industrialized societies by:

too much animal fat in the diet;
too much processed or heated fat;
too much sugar, too much alcohol;
lack of catalysts such as zinc (fertilizers rob the soil of zinc).

**Hypothalamus**
The hypothalamus is situated deep in the brain. Weighing only 4 grams, it is the control centre for food intake, water balance, the autonomic nervous sytem and endocrine levels. The hypothalamus can secrete as many releasing hormones as there are hormones secreted by the anterior pituitary gland. It synthesizes oxytocin and vasopressin, the hormones which are released by the posterior pituitary gland. Since we now know that the hypothalamus can secrete neurohormones, it can be considered to be both an endocrine gland and a part of the brain. This means that there is no longer any frontier between the hormonal system and the nervous system. The hypothalamus can thus be regarded as the orchestrator of the primal adaptive system.

**Lymphocytes**
These are white cells with one nucleus. They are formed in the bone marrow. Those which subsequently mature in the bone marrow and which produce antibodies are called B lymphocytes. Other lymphocytes mature in the thymus

161

and are called T lymphocytes or T cells. T cells are special-ized: T killers can destroy cells; T helpers help B lympho-cytes secrete antibodies; T suppressors reduce the activity of B lymphocytes. Cortisol can destroy 95 per cent of the lymphocytes in the thymus.

## Pineal Gland (or pineal body, or epiphysis)

This is a small reddish-grey structure about the size of a pea situated deep in the brain. Descartes considered it as the centre of the soul. It is only recently that we began to understand its functions.

The pineal gland synthesizes and secretes melatonin. This hormone is secreted all through life, according to a circadian rhythm. Regardless of the sex, the concentrations of circulating hormone are high during the night and low during the day. Eleven days are needed after jet-lag in order to readjust the rhythm of the pineal gland. The night-time secretion of melatonin pulsates, peaking every ten minutes, the highest peak occurring in the middle of the night. Melatonin helps to induce sleep. It has been shown to have an inhibitory effect on numerous hormonal functions.

Melatonin plays an important role in the metabolic pathway of the unsaturated fatty acids and especially in the mobilization of the direct precursor of prostaglandins 1 and in the feedback relationship between the different prosta-glandins. Pineal insufficiency or disturbances in the secretion of melatonin might play an important role in many aspects of *the* disease of civilization. Seasonal depressions and psoriasis are connected with low secretions of melatonin. People with these conditions are badly adapted to darkness: therapies using light seem to work. Colchicine is a drug which imitates the action of melatonin.

Our current knowledge about the pineal gland and mela-tonin suggests that we should be careful not to disturb the

light-dark rhythm at the beginning of life, when the pineal
gland is reaching its set point levels.

## Primal Adaptive System
The primal brain, the hormonal system and the immune
system make up one whole – the primal adaptive system.

## Primal Brain
This is the most ancient part of the brain both in the history
of life and in the history of the individual. It is that part
of the brain which we have in common with all the
mammals. All the structures which have a close relationship
with the hypothalamus belong to the primal brain:
thalamus, hippocampus, amygdala, a rim of cortical structures called limbic system.

## Primal Period
This is the time when a human being is completely dependent on its mother. It includes fetal life, the time of childbirth and the period of breastfeeding. It is the time when
the primal adaptive system reaches its maturity.

## Prostaglandins
Prostaglandins regulate every cell in the body and can be
found in every organ. They are called prostaglandins
because the scientist who discovered them first in 1936
thought they came from the prostate gland. They work on
a second-by-second basis, and their life is short-lived. They
are derived from unsaturated fatty acids. There are three
series of prostaglandins, each derived from a particular
unsaturated fatty acid:

series 1 from dihommogamma linolenic acid;
series 2 from arachidonic acid;
series 3 from eicosapentenoic acid.

Prostaglandins 1 bring about dilation of small vessels and

163

lower the blood pressure. They inhibit the aggregation of platelets, thereby preventing thrombosis. They inhibit the synthesis of cholesterol. They reduce the inflammatory reactions and play an important role in the function of the T lymphocytes.

Prostaglandins 2 play an important role in the process of inflammation. There are important feedback relationships between series 1 and series 2. Corticosteroids, aspirin, non-steroidal anti-inflammatory drugs inhibit the synthesis of series 2 and also of series 1. Some varieties of prostaglandins 2 are commonly used in obstetrics for induction of labour. Not enough is yet known about prostaglandins 3 to make any definite statement about their function.

**Set Point Level**
The set point level can be compared with a domestic thermostat for central heating which is set at a particular temperature or point level. In the body I refer to set point level in connection with the hormonal system. There is a basic hormonal state which is permanently maintained or recovered to its set point level by a feedback mechanism. For example, when the adrenal gland secretes too much cortisol by the standards of the set point level, the high rate of cortisol will reduce the secretion of hormones by the hypothalamus, which will reduce the activity of the pituitary gland and indirectly the activity of the adrenal gland. The level of cortisol will then return to its set point level. What is important is the time when set point levels are established – at the beginning of life. The danger is that when there is an imbalance of the hormones during this critical time the set point level switches can be set too high or too low and thus the hormonal imbalance persists.

**Thymus**
This is a ductless gland situated just behind the top of the breastbone. It is relatively large at birth and gradually

gets smaller after puberty. It is only recently that we have understood its functions. We now know that the thymus plays a key role in the function of T lymphocytes. It is the place where these cells develop their particular specialities. In experiments on animals, when the thymus is taken out immediately after birth, the animal dies. The consequences of the same operation are less spectacular later in life. Situations which knock out the activity of the thymus (high level of cortisol) are probably much more harmful during infancy than later in life. In other words situations of helplessness or hopelessness are especially harmful at the beginning of life.

# Bibliography

CHAPTER 1

Seligman, M. and Weiss, J. 'Coping Behavior: Learned Helplessness, Physiological Change and Learned Inactivity', *Behav Res and Therapy*, 18 (1980) pp. 459–512.

Laborit, H., *L'inhibition de l'action*, Masson, (1980).

Anisman, H.; Remington, G.; Sklar, L., 'Effects of inescapable shock on subsequent escape performance: catecholaminergic and cholinergic mediation of response initiation and maintenance', *Psychopharmacology*, 61 (1979) pp. 107–24.

Cassens, G.; Roffman, M.; Kurne, A.; Orsulak, P.J.; Schildkrant, J., 'Alterations in brain norepinephrine metabolism induced by environmental stimuli previously paired with inescapable shocks', *Science*, 209 (1980) pp. 1138–40.

Lauderslager, M.L.; Ryan, S.M.; Drygan, R.C.; Hyson, R.L.; Maier, S.F., 'Coping and Immunosuppression: Inescapable but not Escapable Shock Suppresses Lymphocyte Proliferation', *Science*, 221 (1983) pp. 568–70.

Visintainer, M.; Volpicelli, J.R.; Seligman, M.E.P., 'Tumor rejection in rats after inescapable or escapable shock', *Science*, 215 (1982) pp. 437–9.

Montaigne; *Essais*, vol, II, p. 37.

Solomon, G.F.; Levine, S.; Kraft, J.K., 'Early experience and immunity', *Nature* (1968) p. 220.


CHAPTER 2

Mechanic, D., 'Students under stress', *The Free Press* (New York, 1962).

Krieger, D.T., 'Brain peptides: what, where, and why?', *Science*, 222 (1983) pp. 975–85.

Cohen, J.J.; Crnic, L.S., *Glucocorticoids, stress and the immune response in immunopharmacology*, (D.R. Webb, 1982).

Felten, S.Y.; Malone, R.K.; Madura, D.J.; Felten, D.L., 'Sympathetic innervation of the spleen', *Soc. Neurosci.*, 9 (1983) p. 116 (abstract no. 34.6).

Williams, J.M.; Peterson, R.G.; Shea, P.A.; Schmedtje, F.J.; Bauer, D.C.; Felten, D.L., 'Sympathetic innervation of murine thymus and spleen. Evidence for a functional link between the nervous and immune systems', *Brain Res. Bulletin*, 6 (1981) pp. 83–94.

Bullock, K.; Moore, R.Y., 'Thymus gland innervation by brain-stem and Spinal Cord in Mouse and Rat', *American Journal of Anatomy*, 162 (1981) pp. 157–66.

Cross, R.J.; Markesbery, W.R.; Brooks, W.H.; Roszman, T.L., 'Hypothalamic-immune interaction I – the acute effect of anterior hypothalamic lesions on the immune response', *Brain Res. Bulletin*, 196 (1980) pp. 79–87.

Stein, M.; Scheifer, S.J.; Keller, S.E., *Hypothalamic influence on immune response in R. Ader psychoneuroimmunology* (Academic Press, 1981).

Wybran J.; Appelbroom, T.; Family, J.P.; Govoaerts, A., 'Suggestive evidence for receptors for morphine and methionine-enkephalin on normal human blood T-lymphocytes', *Journal of Immunology*, 123 (1979) pp. 1068–70.

Hannapel, E.; Xu, G.; Morgan, J.; Hempstead, J.; Horecker, B.L., 'Thymosine B4: a ubiquitous peptide in rat and mouse tissues', *Proc. Nath.*, Academy of Science 79 (1982) pp. 2172–75.

Rebar, R.W.; Miyake, A.; Low, T.L.V.; Goldstein, A.L., 'Thymosin stimulates secretion of luteinizing hormone-releasing factor', *Science*, 213 (1981) pp. 669–71.

Besedovsky, H.O.; Sorkin, E.; Felix, D.; Hass, H., 'Hypothalamic changes during the immune response', *European Journal of Immunology*, 7 (1977) pp. 325–8.

Besedovsky, H.O.; Del Rey, A.; Sorkin, E.; Da Prada, M.; Burri, R.; Honneger, C., 'The immune response evokes changes in brain noradrenergic neurons', *Science*, 221 (1983) pp. 564–6.

Metalnikov, S., 'Role du système nerveux et des facteurs biologiques et psychiques dans l'Immunité', (Masson, 1934).

Ader, R.; Cohen, N., 'Conditioned immunopharmalogical Responses', in *Ader Psychoneuroimmunology* (Academic Press, 1981).

Gorcznski, R.M.; Macrae, S.; Kennedy, M., 'Conditioned immune response associated with allergenic skin grafts in mice', *Journal of Immunology*, 129 (1982) pp. 704–9.

Renoux, G., 'Influence of the brain neocortex on immunity', First International Workshop on Neuroimmunomodulation (Bethesda, MD., 1984).

Calvo, W., 'The innervation of the bone marrow in laboratory animals', *American Journal of Anatomy* (1968) pp. 123–5.

Ader, R.; Cohen, N.; Grota, L.J., 'Adrenal involvement in conditioned immunosuppression', *International Journal of Immunopharmacology*, 1 (1979) pp. 141–5.

Bartrop, R.W.; Luckhurst, E.; Lazarus, L.; Kiloh, L.G.; Penny, R., 'Depressed lymphocyte function after bereavement', *Lancet*, 1 (1977) pp. 834–6.

Schleifer, S.J.; Keller, S.E.; Camerino, M.; Thornton, J.C.; Stein, M., 'Suppression of lymphocyte stimulation following bereavement', *Journal of the American Medical Association*, 250 (1983) pp. 374–7.

Blalock, J.E., 'The immune system as a sensory organ', *Journal of Immunology*, 132 (no. 3) (1984) pp. 1067–70.

Reite, M.; Harbeck. R.; Hoffman, A., 'Altered cellular immune response following peer separation', *Life Science*, 29 (1981) pp. 1133–6.

Sergeeva, V.E., 'Histotopography of catecholamines in the mammelian thymus', *Bulletin Exp. Biological Medicine* (USSR) 77 (1974) pp. 456–8.

Michio, Kushi., *The Book of Macrobiotics* (Japan Publications, 1977).

Hakin Mohammed Said, *Medicine in China* (Hamdard Foundation, Pakistan rev. ed. 1981).

Saez, J.M.; Bertrand, J.; Ducharme, R.; Collu R., 'Autogenèse du système endocrinien', *Les Editions de l'Inserm* (1983).

Pouletty., 'Médecine et chanson', *Le Concours Médical* (March 1985). p. 1009.

CHAPTER 3

Kopaczewiski, W., 'Le terrain, le microbe et l'etat infectieux: Claude Bernard ou Pasteur?', *Revue Scientifique* (July 1936).

Béchamp, A., 'Microzymes et microbes', *Dentu* (1893).

Vogel, F.; Motulsky, A.G., 'Human genetic', *Springer Verlag* (1982).

Feingold, J., 'Génétique médicale acquisition et perspective', *INSERM* Flammarion (1981).

McLearn, G.E.; De Fries, J.C., *Introduction to behavioral genetics* (Freeman, 1973).

Horrobin, D.F., 'Do Eskimos and salmon-eating Canadian indians have a pattern of essential fatty acid metabolism different from europeans?', Abstract of the second international congress on essential fatty acids, prostaglandins and leukotrienes (London, March 1985).

CHAPTER 4

Fevre M.; Segel, T.; Marks, J.F., 'LH and melatonin secretion patterns in pubertal boys', *J. Clin. Endocrinol. Metab.*, 47 (1979) pp. 1383–6.

Fevre-Montange, M.; Van Cauter, E.; Refetoff, S., 'Effects of jet lag on hormonal patterns II adaptation of melatonin circadian periodicity', *J. Clin. Endocrinol. and Metab.*, 52 (1981) pp. 642–9.

Fevre-Montange, M.; Tourniaire, J.; Estour B.; Bajard, L., '24 hour melatonin secretory pattern in Cushing's Syndrome', *Clin. Endocrinol. Metab.*, 18 (1983) pp. 175–81.

Fevre-Montange, M., 'La Mélatonine', *La Presse Médicale*, 14, no 31 (August 1985) pp. 1659–63.

Horrobin, D.F., *Prostaglandins Physiology, Pharmacology and Chemical Significance* (Eden Press, Montreal, 1978).

Karim, S.M.M.; Sandler, M.; Wilhaus, E.D., 'Distribution of prostaglandins in human tissues', *British Journal of Pharmocology*, 31 (1967) pp. 340–4.

Cormvell, D.G.; Huttner J.J.; Milo, G.E., 'Polyunsaturated fatty acids, vitamin E and the proliferation of aortic smooth muscle cells', *Lipids*, 14 (1979) pp. 194–207.

Horrobin, D.F.; Mtabaji, J.P., Mauku, M.S., 'Physiological cortisol levels block the inhibition of vascular reactivity produced by prolactin', *Endocrinology*, 99 (1976) pp. 406–10.

Sihuan, R.E.; Leone, R.M.; Hooper, R.J.L., 'Melatonin, the pineal gland and human puberty', *Nature*, 282 (1979) pp. 301–3.

Stone, K.J.; Willis, A.L.; Hart, M., 'The metabolism of dihomo-gammalinolenic acid in man', *Lipids,* 14 (1979) pp. 174–180.

Fromkel, T.L.; Rivers, J.P.W., 'The Nutritional and metabolic impact of gamma-linolenic acid on cats deprived of animal lipid', *British Journal of Nutrition,* 39 (1978) pp. 227–31.

Kronfol, Ziad; House, J.D., 'Depression, Cortisol and Immune Function', *Lancet* (May 1984) pp. 1026–7.

Beck, A.; Sethi, B.; Tuthill, R., 'Childhood Bereavement and Adult Depression', *Archives of General Psychiatry,* 9 (1963) pp. 295–302.

Brown, F., 'Depression and Childhood Bereavement', *Journal of Mental Sciences* 107 pp. 755–77.

Munro, A., 'Parental Deprivation in Depressive Patients', *British Journal of Psychiatry,* 112 (1966) pp. 443–57.

Horrobin, D.F., 'A Biochemical Basis for Alcoholism and Alcohol-Induced Damage', *Medical Hypotheses,* 6 (1980) pp. 929–42.

Rotrosen, J.; Mandio, D.; Segarwick, D., 'Biochemical and Behavioral Interactions', *Life Science,* 26 (1980) pp. 1867–76.

Dressler, W.W., *Hypertension and Culture Change* (New York 1982).

Olsson, A.G.; Carlson, L.A., 'Prostaglandin E1 in ischemic peripheral arterial disease', International Prostaglandin Conference (Washington May 1979), abstract p. 89.

Steptor, A.; Melville, D., 'Mental health and hypertension', *Lancet* (August 1984) p. 457.

Abdulla, Y.H.; Hamadah, K., 'Effect of ADP on PGE formation in blood platelets from patients with depression, mania and schizophrenia', *British Journal of Psychiatry,* 127 (1975) pp. 591–5.

Horrobin, D.F., 'Schizophrenia: reconciliation of the dopamine, prostaglandin and opioid concepts: role of the pineal', *Lancet,* 1 (1979) pp. 529–31.

171

Horrobin, D.F., 'Schizophrenia as a prostaglandin deficiency disease', *Lancet* 1 (1977) 936–7.

Watamebe, M.; Funahashi, T.; Suzuki, T.; Nomura, S.; Nakazawa, T.; Noguchi, T.; Tsukada, Y., 'Antithymic antibodies in schizophrenic seta?', *Biological Psychiatry*, 17 (1982) pp. 699–710.

Goldstein, A.L.; Rossio, J.; Koliaskina, G.L.; Emory, L.E.; Overall, J.B.; Thurman, G.B.; Hatchur, J., 'Immunological components in schizophrenia', *Perspectives in Schizophrenia Research* (New York 1980) pp. 249–67.

James, W.P.T.; Trayhurn, P., 'Thermogenesis and obesity', *British Medical Bulletin*, 37 (1981) pp. 43–8.

Beardall, Sheila, 'Today's children: fatter, sicker and more disturbed', *The Times* (11 September, 1985).

Zurier, R.B.; Quagliata, F., 'Effect of prostaglandin E1 on adjuvant arthritis', *Nature*, 234 (1971) pp. 304–5.

Taub, S.J.; Zakou, S.J., 'Use of unsaturated fatty acids in the treatment of eczema', *Journal of the American Medical Association*, 105 (1935) pp. 1675.

Gruskay, Frank, 'Comparison of breast, cow, and soy feedings in the prevention of onset of allergic disease', *Clinical Pediatrics* (1982) pp. 486–91.

Glaser, J.; Johnstone, D.F., 'Prophylaxis of allergic disease in the newborn', *JAMA*, 153 (1953) pp. 620.

Johnstone, D.E.; Dutton, A.M., 'Dietary prophylaxis of allergic disease in children', *N.Engl. J. Med.*, 274 (1966) p. 715.

Hamburger, R.; Orgel, M.A., 'The prophylaxis of allergy in infants', *Pediatr. Res.*, 10 (1976) p. 387.

Brown, E.B.; Josephson, B.M.; Levine, H.S., 'A prospective study of allergy in a pediatric population', *Am. J. Dis. Child*, 117 (1969) p. 693.

Halpern, S.R.; Sellar, W.A.; Johnson, R.B., 'Development of

childhood allergy in infants fed breast, soy or cow's milk', *J. Allergy Clin. Immunol.*, 51 (1973) p. 139.

Blaic, H., 'The incidence of asthma, hay fever and infantile eczema in an east Indian group practice of 9145 patients', *Clin. Allergy*, 4 (1974) p. 389.

Van Arsdel, P.P.; Motulaky, A.G., 'Frequency of heritability of asthma and allergic rhinitis in college students', *Acta Genet*, 9 (1959) p. 101.

Grulee, C.G.; Sanford, H.N., 'Influence of breast and artificial feeding on infantile eczema', *J. Pediat*, 9 (1936) p. 223.

Mueller I.I.L.; Weiss, R.J.; O'Lear, D.; Murray, A.E., 'The incidence of milk sensitivity and the development of allergy in infants', *N. Engl. J. Med.*, 268 (1963) p. 1220.

Easthan, E.J.; Lichanco, T.; Grady, M.I., 'Antigenicity of infant formulas: role of immature intestine in protein permeability', *J. Pediatr.*, 93 (1978) p. 561.

Saarinen, U.M.; Bachman, A.; Kajosaari, M., 'Prolonged breastfeeding as prophylaxis for atopic disease', *Lancet*, 2 (1979) p. 163.

Kramer, M.S.; Moroz, B., 'Do breastfeeding and delayed introduction of solid foods protect against subsequent atopic eczema', *J. Pediatr.*, 98 (1981) p. 546.

Davies, T.F. (ed.), *Autoimmune Endocrine Disease* (John Wiley and Sons, 1983).

Saxon, A.; Stevens, R.H.; Ramer, S.J.; Clements, P.; Yu, D.T., 'Glucocorticoids administered in vitro inhibit human suppressor T lymphocyte function and diminish B lymphocyte responsiveness in vitro immunoglobulin synthesis', *Journal of Clinical Investigation*, 61, no 4 (1978) pp. 922–30.

Gallagher, T.F.; Hellman, L.; Finkelstein, J., 'Hyperthyroidism and cortisol secretion in man', *Journal of Clinical Endocrinology Metab.* 34: no. 6 (1972) pp. 919–27.

Aoki, N.; Pinnamanini, K.M.; De Groot L.J., 'Studies on

suppressor cell function in thyroid diseases', *Journal of Clinical Endocrinology Metab.*, 48, no 5 (1979) pp. 803–10.

Meyer, O.; Cyna, L.; Haim, T.; Ryckewoert, A., 'Les anticorps antihistone de type IgG. Valeur diagnostique au cours de la polyarthrite rhumatoide, de la sclérodemie, de la maladie lupique spontanée et medicamenteuse', *Revue Rhum.*, 51 (1984) pp. 303–10.

Diaz, A.; Glamb, R.W.; Silva, J. Jr., 'A syndrome of multiple immune autoreactivity: a breakdown in immune regulation', *Archives Dermatology*, 116 (1980) pp. 77–9.

Bottazzo, G.F.; Florin-Christiensen, A.; Doniach, D., 'Islet-cell antibodies in diabetes mellitus with autoimmune polyendocrine deficiencies', *Lancet*, 2 (1974) pp. 1279–82.

Backkeskov, S.; Nielsen, J.J.; Horner, B.; Bilde, T.; Ludvigsson, J.; Lernmerk. A., 'Autoantibodies in newly diagnosed diabetic children immuno-precipitate human islet-cell proteins', *Nature*, 298 (1982) pp. 167–9.

Minick, C.R.; Fabricant, C.G.; Fabricant, J., 'Atheroarteriosclerosis induced by infection with a herpes virus', *American Journal of Pathology*, 96 (1979) pp. 673–706.

Enig, M.G.; Munn, R.J.; Kenney, M., 'Dietary fat and cancer trends', *Fed. Proc*, 37 (1978) pp. 2215–20.

Van der Merve, C.F.; Boojens, J., 'Gamma linolenic acid in the treatment of primary liver cancer', *Abstracts of the Second International Congress on Essential Fatty Acids, Prostaglandins and Leukotriens* (March 1985).

Costa, D.; Mestes, E.; Coban, A., 'Breast and other cancer deaths in a mental hospital', *Neoplasma*, 181–28, pp. 371–8.

Biran, N.; Schloot, W., 'Pathological nychthemeral rhythm of melatonin secretion in psoriasis', *IRCS Journal of Medical Science*, 7 (1979) p. 400.

174

# CHAPTER 5

Klaus, M.; Kennel, J., *Parent-Infant Bonding*, (Mosby, 1982).

Rosenblatt, J.S., 'Progress in the study of maternal behavior in animals', in Klaus, M. and Robertson M.O., *Birth Interaction and Attachment* (Johnson and Johnson, 1982).

Rosenblatt, J.S., 'Nonhormonal basis of maternal behavior', *Science*, 156 (1967) pp. 1512–4.

Dörner, G., *Hormones and Brain Differentiation* (Amsterdam, 1976).

Dörner, G.; Standt, J., 'Perinatal structural sex differentiation of the hypothalamus in rats', *Neuroendocrinology* 5 (1969) pp. 103–6.

Goy, Robert, McEwen, Bruce, *Sexual Differentiation of the Brain*, (Cambridge, Mass., 1977).

Dörner, G,; Standt, J., 'Structural changes in the hypothalamic ventromedial nucleus of the male rat following neocortal castration and androgen treatment', *Neuroendocrinology*, 4 (1969) pp. 278–81.

Dörner G.; Hinz, G.; Döcke, F.; Tönjes, R., 'Effects of psychotrophic drugs on brain differentiation in female rats', *Endokrinologie*, 70 (1977) pp. 113–23.

Dörner, G.; Rohde, W.; Stahl, F.; Krell, L.; and Masius, W.G., 'A neuroendocrine predisposition for homosexuality in men', *Arch. Sex. Behav.*, 4 (1975) pp. 1–8.

Chaouat, G.; Kolb, J.P.; Wegmann, T.G., 'The murine placenta as an immunological barrier between the mother and the fetus', *Immunology Review*, 75 (1983) pp. 31–60.

Sony, J.; Clot, J.; Bouman, M.; Andary, M., 'Immunomodulating effect of human placenta eluted gammaglobulines in rheumatoid arthritis', *Arthritis Rheumatology*, 25 (1982) p.17.

Benhamon, C.L.; Brandeley, M., 'Influence de la grossesse et de l'etat hormonal sur la polyarthrite rhumatoide', *La Presse Médicale* (15 October 1983), 12, no.36 pp. 2223–4.

Voisin, G.A.; Chaouat, G., 'Demonstration, nature and properties of antibodies fixed on maternal placenta and directed against paternal antigens', *Journal of Reproduction and Fertility*, 21 (1974) pp. 89–103.

Chard, T.; Hudson, C.N.; Edwards, C.R.W.; Boyd, N.R.H., 'Release of oxytocin and vasopressin by the human fetus during labor', *Nature*, 234 pp. 352–4.

CHAPTER 6

Welin, L.; Svärdsudd, L.; Ander-Peciva, S.; Tibblin, G.; Tibblin, B.; Larsson, B.; Wilhelmsen, L., 'Prospective Study of Social Influences on Mortality', *Lancet* (20 April, 1985) pp. 915–8.

Cassel, J., 'The contribution of the social environment to host resistance', *American Journal of Epidemiology*, 104 (1976) pp. 107–23.

House, J.S.; Robbins, C.; Mentzner, H.L., 'The association of social relationships and activities with mortality: prospective evidence for the tecumseh community health study', *American Journal of Epidemiology*, 116 (1982) pp. 123–140.

Berkman, L.F.; Syme, S.L., 'Social networks, host resistance, and mortality: a nine-year follow-up study of almeda county residents', *American Journal of Epidemiology*, 109 (1979) pp. 186–204.

CHAPTER 7

Mansfield, Peter, *Common Sense About Health* (Templegarth Trust, 1982).

Mansfield, Peter; 'Neighborhood health cultivation service in soil, food and health in a changing world', Proceedings of the McCarrison Society Conference (July, 1980).

Cousins, Norman; *Anatomy of an Illness* (Norton, 1979).

Benson, H., 'The placebo effects: a neglected asset in the care of patients', *Journal of the American Medical Association*, 232 (12 June 1975).

Shapiro, A.K., 'Placebo effects in psychotherapy and psychanalysis', *Journal of Clinical Pharmacology*, 10 (1970) pp. 73–8.

'Le Vieux Cognet', *Art et Thérapie – Revue Mensuelle*, Levée des Grouëts, 41000 Blois.

Graham, J.; *Multiple Sclerosis: A Self-Help Guide to its Management* (Thorsons, 1981).

Eaton, B.; Konner, M.; 'Paleolithic nutrition', *The New England Journal of Medicine*, 312–5, pp. 283–99.

Kay, R.; 'Diets of early miocene African hominoids', *Nature*, 268 (1977) pp. 628–30.

Draper, H.H., 'The aboriginal eskimo diet in modern perspective', *American Anthropology*, 79 (1977) pp. 309–16.

Crawford, M.A., 'Fatty-acid ratios in free-living and domestic animals', *Lancet* 1 (1968) pp. 1329–33.

Moncada, E.S.; Vane, J.R., 'Eicosapentaenoic acid and prevention of thrombosis and atherosclerosis', *Lancet*, 2 (1978) pp. 117–9.

Sinclair, H.M., 'Essential fatty acids in perspective', *Human Nutrition Chemical Nutrition*, 38C (1984) pp. 245–60.

Graham, J.; *Evening Primrose Oil* (Thorsons, 1984).

CHAPTER 8

'High technology medicine: a luxury we can afford', *Lancet* (July 1984) pp. 77–8.

Escoffier-Lambiotte, 'Un Rapport sur l'evaluation des techniques et des pratiques médicales', *Le Monde* (28 June 1985).

Frendenheim, M., 'Business and Health', *The New York Times* (11 June 1985).

Weitz, M.; *Health Shock* (David and Charles, 1980).

'The hazards intravenous therapy', *New England Journal of Medicine*, 294, pp. 1178–1976.

Herbst A., 'Diethylstilbestrol exposure', *New England Journal of Medicine*, 311 (1984) pp. 1433–4.

Greenberg, E.R.; Bernes, A.; Ressegule, L., 'Breast cancer in mothers given diethylstilbestrol in pregnancy', *New England Journal of Medecine*, 311 (1984) 1393–8.

Shuman, R., 'Neurotoxicity of hexachlorophane in the human', *Journal of Pediatrics*, 54 (1974) p. 689.

Taylor, D.W.; Haynes, R.B.; Sackett, D.H., 'Long-term followup of abstenteism among working men following the detection and treatment of their hypertension', *Clin. Invest. Med.*, 4 (1981) pp. 173–7.

Mouk, M., 'Blood pressure awareness and psychological well-being in the health and nutrition examination survey', *Clin. Invest. Med.* 4 (1981) pp. 183–90.

Soghikian, K.; Fallick-Hunkeler, E.M.; Vri, H.K.; Fisher, A.A., 'The effect of high blood pressure awareness and treatment on emotional well-being', *Clin. Invest. Med.*, 4 (1981) pp. 191–6.

Steptoe, A.; Melville, D., 'Mental Health and Hypertension', *Lancet*, (25 August, 1984) p. 457.

Béchamp, A., 'Sur la préparation et les caractères du sous nitrate de bismuth,' avec C. Saintpierre, *Montpellier Médical*. (1860).

Olivier, R.; Hetzel, B., 'Rise and fall of suicide rates in Australia: relation to sedative availability', *Medical Journal* 2 (August 1972) p. 919.

Nightingale, S., 'Inappropriate prescribing of psychoactive drugs', *Ann. Int. Med.*, 83 (1975) pp. 896–975.

Skolnick, P.; Paul S.M., 'Benzodiazephine receptors', *Annual Reports in Medicinal Chemistry* (Academic Press, 1981).

Ruff, M.; Pert, C.; Weber, R.; Wahl, L.; Wahl, S.; Paul, S.,

'Benzodiazepine receptor-mediated chemotaxis of human monocytes', *Science*, 299 (1985) pp. 1281–3.

Hemminki, E., 'Diuretics in pregnancy: a case study of a worthless therapy', *Social Science Medicine*, 18, no 12 (1984) pp. 1011–8.

'Cyclosporin in auto-immune disease', *Lancet* (April 1985) pp. 909–11.

Read, J., 'The reported increase in mortality from asthma. A clinical-functional analysis', *Medical Journal of Australia*, 1 (1968) p. 879.

'Antibiotic resistance and topical treatment', *British Medical Journal*, 2 (1978) p. 649.

Altemeier, W., 'Changing patterns in surgical infections', *American Surgery*, 178 (1973) p. 436.

Vayda, E., 'A comparison of surgical notes in Canada and in England and Wales', *N. Engl. Journal of Medicine* 289 (1973) p. 1224.

Vernin P.H.; Bonneterre, Demaille, A., 'Les cancers induits par la chirurgie existent-ils?', *Le Concours Médical* (March 1985) pp. 107–11.

Turunen, M.J.; Klvilaakso, E.V., 'Increasing risk of colorectal cancer after cholecystectomy', *Ann. Surgery*, 195 (1981) pp. 639–41.

Dougherty, S.H.; Foster, C.A.; Eisenberg, M.M., 'Stomach cancer following gastric surgery for benign disease,' *Arch. Surg.*, 117 (1982) pp. 295–7.

'Surgery for coronary artery disease', *British Medical Journal*, 1 (1978) p. 597.

Glicksman, A., 'Malignant radiation of benign conditions', *Ann. International Medicine*, 89 (1978) p. 130.

Peterson, O., 'Myocardial infarction: unit care or home care?', *Ann. Int. Med.*, 88 (1978) p. 259.

Mather, H., 'Myocardial infarction: a comparison between home and hospital care for patients', *British Medical Journal*, 1 (1976) p. 925.

Hill, J., 'Comparison of mortality of patients with heart attacks admitted to a coronary care unit and an ordinary medical ward', *British Medical Journal*, 2 (1977) p. 81.

Bailar, J., 'Mammography: a contrary view', *Ann. Int. Med.*, 84 (1976) p. 77.

Adams, D., 'Complications of coronary angiography', *Cire*, 48 (1973) p. 609.

Mubroy, R., 'Iatrogenic disease in general practice: its incidence and effects', *British Medical Journal*, 2 (1973) p. 407.


CHAPTER 9


Salk, L.; Sturner, W.Q.; Lipsitt, L.P.; Reilly, B.M.; Levat, R.H., 'Relationship of maternal and perinatal conditions to eventual adolescent suicide', *Lancet* (March 1985) pp. 625–7.

Borch-Johnsen, K.; Mandrup-Poulsen, T.; Zachau-Christiansen, B.; Geir, J.; Christy, M.; Kestrup, K.; Nerup, J.; 'Relation between breastfeeding and incidence rates of insulin-dependant diabetes mellitus', *Lancet* (November 1984) pp. 1083–6.

Groen, J.J., 'Psychosomatic aspects of meniere's disease', *Acta Otolaryngology* 95 (1983) pp. 407–16.

Ronne, T., 'Measles virus infection without rash in childhood is related to disease in adult life', *Lancet* (January 1985) 8419.

Sobrinho, L.G.; Nunes, M.C.P.; Calhaz-Jorge, C., 'Hyperprolactinemia in women with paternal deprivation during childhood', *Obstetric Gynaecology*, 64–4 (1984) pp. 465–8.

Daling, J. 'Birth weight and the incidence of childhood cancer', *Journal of the National Cancer Institute*, 72, 5 pp. 1039–41.

Tinbergen, N. and E., *Autistic Children: New Hope for a Cure* (London, 1983).

Illsley, R.; Mitchel, R.; *Low Birth Weight: A Medical, Psychological and Social Study* (John Wiley and Sons, 1984).

Marmot, M.G.; Paye, C.M.; Atkins, E., 'Effects of breastfeeding on plasma cholesterol and weight in young adults', *Journal of Epidemiology Community Health*, 34 (1980) pp.164–7.

Geschwind, N.; Behan, P., 'Left-handedness: association with immune disease, migraine and developmental learning disorder', *Proc. National Academy of Science*, 79 (1982) pp.5097–6000.

Nicol, A.R., *Longitudinal Studies in Child Psychology and Psychiatry* (John Wiley, 1985).

Butler, N.R.; Corner, B.D., 'Stress and disability in childhood – the long-term problems', *Proceedings of the Thirty-fourth Symposium of the Colston Research Society* (March 1982).

Wadsworth, M.E., 'Delinquency, pulse rates and early emotional deprivation in a national sample of children', *British Journal of Criminology*, 316 (1976) pp. 145–56.

Menkes, J.J., 'Early feeding history of children with learning disorders', *Developmental Medicine and Child Neurology*, 19, pp. 169–71.

Rodgers, B., 'Feeding in infancy and later ability and attainment: a longitudinal study', *Developmental Medicine and Child Neurology*, 20 no.4 (August, 1978) pp. 421–6.

CHAPTER 10

Haire, D., *The Cultural Warping of Childbirth*, ICEA 251 (Nottingham Way Hillside, NJ., 1972).

Donnison, J., *Midwives and Medical Men* (Heinemann, 1977).

Illich, I., *Medical Nemesis* (Pantheon, 1976).

Kitzinger, S., *The Experience of Childbirth* (Penguin, 1976).

Kitzinger, S., *Birth At Home* (Oxford University Press, 1979).

Junor, V.; Monaco, M., *Home Birth* (Souvenir, 1984).

Noble, E., *Childbirth With Insight* (Boston, 1983).

Odent, M.; *Birth Reborn* (New York, 1984).

Odent, M.; *Towards a Less Mechanized Childbirth. Advances in International Maternal and Child Health* (Oxford University Press, 1985).

Arms, S., *Immaculate Deception* (Boston, 1975).

Leboyer, F.; *Pour Une Naissance Sans Violence* (Paris, 1974).

Odent, M.; *Bien Naitre* (Paris, 1976).

Odent, M.; *Genèse de l'homme Ecologique* (Paris, 1979).

Verny, T.; Kelly, J.; *The Secret Life of the Unborn Child* (Summit Books, 1981).

Balaskas, J.; *Active Birth* (Unwin Paperbacks, 1983).

This, B.; *Naitre* (Paris, 1972).

Morley, G.K.; Mooradian, A.; Levine, A.; Morley, J., 'Mechanism of pain in diabetic peripheral neuropathy', *American Journal of Medicine*, 77 (July 1984) pp. 79–82.

Singhi, S.; Chookang, E.; Hall, J.St E.; Kalghatgi, S., 'Iatrogenic neonatal and maternal hyponatraemia following oxytocin and aqueous glucose infusion during labour', *British Journal of Obstetrics and Gynaecology*, 92 (April 1985) pp. 356–63.

Kenepp, N.B.; Shelley, W.C.; Gabbe, S.G.; Kumar, S.; Stanley, C.A.; Gutsche, B.B., 'Fetal and neonatal hazards of maternal hydration with 5% dextrose before caesarean section', *Lancet*, (May 1982) pp. 1150–2.

Singhi, S.; Kang, E.C.; Hall, J.St E., 'Hazards of maternal hydration with 5% Dextrose', *Lancet* (August 1982) pp.335–6.

Lucas, A.; Adrian, T.E.; Aynsley-Green, A.; Bloom, S.R., 'Iatrogenic hyperinsulism at birth', *Lancet* (January 1980).

Milner, R.D.G.; Hales, C.N.; (1965), 'Effect of Intravenous Glucose on Concentration of Insulin in Maternal and Umbilical Cord Plasma', *British Medical Journal* (1965) pp. 284–6.

182

Lawrence G.F.; Brown, V.A.; Parsons, R.J., 'Fetal-maternal consequences of high dose glucose infusion during labor', *Br. J. Obste. Gynecol.*, 89 (1982) pp. 27–32.

Goodfellow, C.F.; Hull, M.G.R.; Swaab, D.F.; Dogterom, J.; Buijs, R.M., 'Oxytocin deficiency at delivery with epidural analgesia', *Br. J. Obste. Gynecol.*, 90 (March 1983) pp. 214–9.

Knobloch, H.; Rider, R.; Harper, R., 'Neuropsychiatric sequelae of prematurity', *Journal of the American Medical Association*, 161 (1956) pp. 53–74.

Tuck, S.J.; Monin, P.; Duvivier, C.D.; May, T.; Vert, P., 'Effect of a rocking bed on apnoea of prematurity', *Arch. Dis. Child* 57 (1982) pp. 475–7.

Rice, R., 'Neurophysiological development in premature infants following stimulation', *Developmental Psychology*, 13(1) (1977) pp. 69–76.

Ludington, S.M., 'Vaginal and cesarean delivered infants' response to extra tactile stimulation', Thesis (Texas Women's University, Denton, May 1977).

Jonscis, J.H.P., 'A premature's nursery without incubators', *Acta Paediatrica Scandinavia*, Supplement 172 (1967) pp. 100–2.

CHAPTER 11

Newton, N., *Family Book of Child Care* (New York, 1957).

Montagu, A., *Touching* (New York, 1971).

Salk, L., *What Every Child Would Like His Parents to Know* (New York, 1972).

Gay, L.; Segal, J., *Insomnia* (New York, 1969).

La Leche League International (1958), *The Womanly Art of Breastfeeding*, 9116 Minneapolis Avenue Franklin Park; II.

Prescott, J.W., *Cross Cultural Studies*, HEW, Growth and Development Branch, National Institute of Child Health and Human Development, Bethesda, MD.

Thevenin, T., *The Family Bed* (Minneapolis, 1976).

Stanway, P. and A., *Breast Is Best* (Pan, 1983).

Kitzinger, S., *The Experience of Breastfeeding* (Penguin, 1970).

Prescott, J., 'Body pleasure and the origin of violence', *The Futurist*, 9(2) (1975) pp. 64–74.

Rice, R., 'Infant stress and the relationship to violent behavior', *Neonatal Network* (April, 1985).

Bury, B., *The Idea of Progress* (Macmillan, 1932).

### HISTORICAL NOTE

Vallery-Radot, R., *La Vie de Pasteur* (Paris, 1911).

Dubos, R., *Louis Pasteur, Franc Tireur de la Science* (Paris, 1950).

Hume, E.D., *Béchamp ou Pasteur? Un Chapitre Perdu de la Biologie* (Paris, 1948).

Decourt, Philippe, 'Béchamp et Pasteur', *Archives International Claude Bernard* (October 1971).

Latour, B., *Les Microbes – Guerre et Paix* (Paris, 1984).

Béchamp, A., *Les Microzymas dans leurs Rapports avec L'hétérogonie, L'histogonie, la Physiologie et La Pathologie* (Paris, 1883).

Nonclercq, M.; *Béchamp, A., L'homme et le Savant Originalité et Fécondité de son Oeuvre* (Paris, 1982).

Nonclercq, M., *Un Inconnu: Le Professeur Antoine Béchamp* (Cercle des Amis, Bordeaux, 1975).

Nonclercq, M., 'Une Injustice Dans L'Historie des Sciences', *Bulletin Ac. et Ste Lorraines des Sciences* 4 (1977) pp. 137–61.

Nonclercq, M., 'Un Chapitre Ignoré de L'Histoire des Sciences.

L'Oeuvre de Béchamp', Fasc. V 103ème Congrès des Sociétés Savantes (Nancy, 1978).

# Index

'A' blood group, 35
Acid(s):
 amino, 96, 123
 fatty, 33, 41, 44, 54, 69, 72–3,
  96–8, 160
 gamma-linolenic, 44, 51, 54,
  72, 97, 99, 111, 161
 linoleic, 44
 monounsaturated fatty, 160
 polyunsaturated fatty, 97, 160
 unsaturated fatty, 33, 41, 55,
  162
Acquired Immune Deficiency
  Syndrome
  (AIDS), 19, 31–2, 53, 111,
  119
ACTH, 24, 28, 61, 158
Additives, food, 50
Adrenal:
 glands, 23, 24, 41, 52, 64, 112
 hormones, 55
Adrenalin, 11, 58, 68, 103, 134,
  158
Ageing, 43, 54–5
Agriculture, 76, 96–8
AIDS, 19, 31–2, 53, 111, 119
Alcohol(ism), 39, 44, 46, 87, 95,
  98
Allergy(ies), 21, 37, 39, 49–51,
  53, 105, 123
 food, 50, 128
Amino acids, 96, 123
Angioplasty, 114
Animal(s):
 behaviour, 59
 experiments on, 10, 25, 54, 60,
  82
 fat, 31, 111
Antibiotics, 71, 101, 109, 117
Antibodies:
 IgA, 29, 51, 72, 95
 IgG, 29

IgM, 28–9
Antigens, 24, 35, 51
Art, 79, 80, 84–8
 healing and, 84
 therapy, 87, 88
Arteriosclerosis, 96
Arthritis, rheumatoid, 52, 111
Aspirin, 105, 129, 164
Attachment, 59–62, 121
Aucher, Marie Louise, 86–7
Autistic children, 126–7
Auto-immune diseases, 21, 39,
  51–3, 111

Baby(ies):
 carriers, 147
 comparisons between, 37
 separated from mother, 9, 36,
  40–1, 42, 43, 50, 51, 67,
  126, 143, 144, 147–9
 sleeping with mother, 147–9
Bacteria, 11, 19–20, 21, 28, 29,
  70–1, 82–3, 95, 101–2, 121,
  122, 144
'B' lymphocyte, 20
Béchamp, Antoine, 32, 121,
  154–7
Behaviour:
 animal, 59
 anti-social, 76
 maternal, 23, 59–60
 sexual, 27, 62–6
 submissive, 11
Behavioural disorders, 46, 107
Behavioural response, 11
Birth:
 home, 132–3, 136, 146, 150
 multiple, 110
 presence of father at, 136,
  137–41, 142
 privacy at, 138–43
 rate reduction, 131

187

Multiple births, 110
Multiple sclerosis, 53, 111
Muscle(s), 52
  pain, 50
  weakness, 35
Music, 86, 87
  therapy, 87

Neocortex, 19, 29–30, 68, 79, 90,
  128, 139
Neonatology, 143–5, 146
Nerve(s), 24, 103
  cells, 15, 22, 23, 25, 27, 46, 65
  optic, 27
Nervous system, 11, 14, 18, 25,
  64
Newborn babies:
  medicine of, 143–5
  separation from mother, 9, 36,
    40–1, 42, 43, 50, 51, 67,
    126, 143, 144, 147–9
New brain, 19, 29–30, 68
Noradrenalin, 24, 43, 158
Nuclear:
  family, 90, 130–2, 146, 150
  war, 53
Nutrition, 10, 13, 94, 98

Obesity, 36, 39, 47–8
'O' blood group, 35
Obstetrics, 66, 68, 125, 132–8,
  143, 146, 150, 164
Oesophagus, cancer of, 54
Oestrogen, 23, 59, 63, 101
Orgasm, 62, 80
Oriental medicine, 25
Oxytocin, 23, 65, 68, 161

Pasteur, Louis, 25, 31, 32, 82,
  121, 153–7
Penicillin, 109
Phagocytes, 20, 28
Pineal gland, 41, 43, 47, 52, 124,
  162–3
Pituitary:
  gland, 22, 28, 55
  hormones, 22, 28, 63
  oxytocin, 23, 65
Plague, 32, 85, 86
Pollution, 95
Polyunsaturated fatty acid, 97
Potassium, 103

Pregnancy, 63–9, 76–7, 92,
  130–1
  and drugs, 101, 105, 108, 115
  mystery surrounding, 65–6,
    140, 142
Primal adaptive system, 15–16,
  18–30, 39, 41, 55, 58, 62,
  65–6, 68–9, 83, 94, 98, 112,
  163
Primal brain, 14–16, 22, 55, 79,
  83, 151, 163
  early development of, 26–30
Primal health centres, 149–52
Prise de conscience, 109, 130–45
Privacy in childbirth, 138–43
Procreation, 57–9, 74
Progesterone, 23, 65, 69
Prolactin, 47, 59, 69, 81
Prostaglandins, 41–2, 44, 47–56,
  65, 96, 98, 107, 134, 162–4
  1, 41–4, 46–56, 68, 69, 72, 97,
    105, 162
  2, 41–2, 48, 56, 68, 105
  3, 41
Proteins, 23, 49, 51, 95, 96, 97,
  107
Psoriasis, 123–4
Puberty, 21, 124

Questions on health, 32–3

Rabelais, 88, 104
Reducing birth rate, 131
Religion, 74–81, 87
Research:
  on autistic children, 126–7
  long-term, 125, 127–8
  money in, 118–19
  new kinds of, 128–9
  in primal health, 118–29, 157
  short-term, 125–6
Responses, behavioural, 11
Rheumatism, 39, 48, 104–6,
  119
Rheumatoid arthritis, 52, 111

Saturated fats, 97, 98
Schizophrenia, 36, 39, 46–7
Seasonal depression, 43
Sensory:
  functions, 16, 84, 94, 122
  organs, 16, 26, 29

191